OANL

OXFORD AMERICAN NEUROLOGY LIBRARY

Sleep Disorders

The Clinician's Guide to Diagnosis and Management

D1546396

O A N L
OXFORD AMERICAN NEUROLOGY LIBRARY

Sleep Disorders

The Clinician's Guide to Diagnosis and Management

Ruth M. Benca, MD, PhD

Director, Center for Sleep Medicine and Sleep Research
Professor, Department of Psychiatry
University of Wisconsin School of Medicine and Public Health
Madison, WI

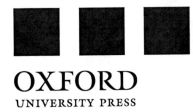

OXFORD
UNIVERSITY PRESS

OXFORD
UNIVERSITY PRESS

Oxford University Press, Inc., publishes works that further
Oxford University's objective of excellence
in research, scholarship, and education.

Oxford New York

Auckland Cape Town Dar es Salaam Hong Kong Karachi
Kuala Lumpur Madrid Melbourne Mexico City Nairobi
New Delhi Shanghai Taipei Toronto

With offices in
Argentina Austria Brazil Chile Czech Republic France Greece
Guatemala Hungary Italy Japan Poland Portugal Singapore
South Korea Switzerland Thailand Turkey Ukraine Vietnam

Published by Oxford University Press, Inc.
198 Madison Avenue, New York, New York 10016
www.oup.com

Oxford is a registered trademark of Oxford University Press

Library of Congress Cataloging-in-Publication Data

Benca, Ruth Myra,
Sleep disorders : the clinician's guide to diagnosis and management / Ruth Benca.
p. ; cm. -- (Oxford American neurology library)
Includes bibliographical references and index.
ISBN 978-0-19-538973-9 (pbk. : alk. paper)
1. Sleep disorders—Diagnosis. 2. Sleep disorders—Treatment. I. Title. II. Series:
Oxford American neurology library.
[DNLM: 1. Sleep Disorders—diagnosis. 2. Sleep Disorders—therapy. WM 188]
RC547.B46 2011
616.8'498--dc22   2011012554

Dedication

To Jose, Zulema, Nick and Bart

Disclosures

Dr. Benca has served as a consultant to Merck and Sanofi-aventis.

Preface

Over 50 million people in the United States suffer from chronic disorders of sleep and wakefulness. Sleep disorders and insufficient sleep impact negatively on virtually every medical and psychiatric condition and lead to increased morbidity and mortality. Unfortunately, sleep medicine training for medical professionals is often inadequate. The purpose of this handbook is to help practitioners diagnose and treat common sleep disorders and recognize when referral to a sleep medicine specialist may be needed. Although not intended to replace more comprehensive textbooks in the field, this text should also serve as a useful resource for the sleep medicine specialist.

The book includes chapters on the science of normal sleep and the clinical evaluation of sleep complaints. The epidemiology, diagnosis and treatment of the major categories of sleep disorders are discussed in chapters on insomnia, sleep-related breathing disorders, hypersomnias, circadian rhythm disorders, parasomnias and sleep-related movement disorders. Tables with diagnostic criteria, differential diagnosis of sleep-related symptoms, treatment guidelines and medications are provided in each chapter and are consistent with practice parameters of the American Academy of Sleep Medicine.

I would like to gratefully acknowledge the editorial assistance of Annette Vee in the preparation of this book, as well as thank my colleagues for their careful reviews of the manuscript, helpful suggestions and contributions, including Mary Carskadon, Chiara Cirelli, Clete A. Kushida, Mark W. Mahowald, Charles M. Morin, David T. Plante and James K. Walsh.

Contents

Chapter 1

Normal Sleep

Sleep is a universal behavior that has been demonstrated in every animal studied to date, ranging from insects to humans. Humans spend about one third of their lives sleeping. Insufficient or inadequate sleep, as a result of medical, psychiatric, or sleep disorders or sleep deprivation, can have serious health consequences. Conversely, even normal sleep is accompanied by physiological changes that can affect a variety of medical disorders. Furthermore, many commonly used medications and substances can affect sleep through interactions with systems in the brain that promote sleep or wakefulness. A basic understanding of normal sleep behavior, physiology, and neurobiology is therefore essential for proper diagnosis and treatment of sleep disorders.

What is Sleep?

Sleep is a behavioral state characterized by decreased awareness of the environment, adoption of a characteristic posture with reduced movement (usually lying in bed with eyes closed), and reduced sensitivity to stimuli, distinguishing it from rest. Sleep is usually easily reversible (i.e., a sleeping individual can usually be aroused by increased sensory stimulation), which distinguishes it from other similarly appearing states such as coma or unconsciousness. Normal individuals usually have a fairly good ability to recognize and report their own sleep behavior; we are generally aware that we are sleepy, and although we do not necessarily recall the exact moment of sleep onset, we are usually aware of having gone to sleep and that we have slept, as well as some general sense of the amount of time that we have slept.

Sleep can also be defined by electrophysiological parameters, usually recorded in sleep laboratories for clinical or research purposes. The minimal parameters required to identify sleep and classify its stages include the **electroencephalogram (EEG)**, measurement of eye movements or **electrooculogram (EOG)**, and measurement of muscle activity or **electromyogram (EMG)**. Sleep is usually scored by visual inspection in epochs or segments of 30 seconds across the night according to standardized criteria, originally described by Rechtschaffen and Kales in 1968[1] and modified by the American Academy of Sleep Medicine in 2007[2] (Table 1.1). Stages of sleep and wakefulness are identified through specific EEG waveforms, the presence or absence of eye movements, and level of muscle activity. There are two types of sleep, **rapid eye movement (REM) sleep** and **non-REM (NREM) sleep**. REM sleep is sometimes referred to as dreaming sleep because it is usually accompanied by prominent dreaming. Dreaming can also occur in NREM sleep, although this is less common. NREM sleep is further subdivided into stages N1, N2, and N3. Electrophysiological characteristics of sleep stages are listed in Table 1.1.

Table 1.1 Sleep Stages

Stage Wake (W)

EEG: Low voltage, fast activity. Alpha rhythm (8–12 Hz), most prominent when eyes closed and over occipital regions.

EMG: Variable; higher than during sleep

EOG: Eye blinks, eye movements present

Stage N1 (NREM1)

EEG: 4- to 7-Hz activity, background frequencies slowed in comparison to W. Vertex sharp waves.

EMG: Variable, but lower than stage W

EOG: Slow, rolling eye movements

Stage N2 (NREM2)

EEG: K-complexes (negative sharp waves followed by positive component, total duration >0.5 s) and sleep spindles (11–16 Hz, duration >0.5 s)

EMG: Lower than stage W

EOG: Usually absent

Stage N3 (NREM3)

EEG: Slow waves (0.5–2 Hz) with amplitude >75 μv measured over frontal regions

EMG: Lower than stage N2

EOG: Usually absent

Stage R (REM)

EEG: Low amplitude, mixed frequency. Sawtooth waves (2–6 Hz).

EMG: Predominantly low-absent, with superimposed, brief bursts of increased activity, maximal when accompanying eye movements

EOG: Rapid eye movements

Adapted with permission from the American Academy of Sleep Medicine. *The AASM Manual for the Scoring of Sleep and Associated Events: Rules, Terminology and Technical Specification.* Darien, IL: American Academy of Sleep Medicine; 2007.

During wakefulness, the EEG shows an activated pattern, with low voltage and fast activity. Eye movements, eye blinks, and muscle activity are also present. Just before sleep onset, when an individual is lying in bed with eyes closed, a prominent alpha rhythm (8–13 Hz) typically appears in the EEG. Eye movements and muscle activity are usually decreased.

Individuals normally enter sleep through **stage N1**, which is characterized by the alpha rhythm disappearing and being replaced by a low-voltage mixed-frequency pattern, often with theta (4–7 Hz) activity and occasional vertex sharp waves. Muscle activity is decreased and slow, rolling eye movements are present. Stage N1 is also accompanied by decreased awareness of the environment, with a preferential loss of visual perception, although there may be some continued partial awareness as well as a subjective sense of being awake rather than asleep. Thoughts become more dream-like, and individuals may report dreaming during this stage. Normally, stage N1 is a transition into sleep and occupies a small proportion of sleep time (around 5%).

Stage **N2** typically follows and is characterized by the appearance of sleep spindles, bursts of 11–16-Hz EEG activity lasting at least 0.5 sec, and K-complexes, which are high-amplitude, negative sharp waves followed by positive slow waves. Muscle activity is decreased and eye movements are absent.

Stage **N3** is similar to N2, except that slow waves (0.5–2 Hz with amplitude >75 µV) become more frequent, occupying at least 20% of each epoch; N3 is also referred to as **slow-wave sleep (SWS)**. Both stages N2 and N3 are subjectively perceived as sleep, and the arousal threshold increases progressively across stages N1 to N3. Adults will typically spend about 70% to 75% of the night in stages 2 and 3 combined.

REM sleep **(stage R)** has an activated EEG pattern, similar to stage N1; increased theta activity as well as trains of sawtooth (2–6 Hz, triangular, serrated) waves may be present. The stage takes its name from the fact that irregular bursts of rapid eye movements are seen in the EOG channel. Muscle activity is characterized by a tonic atonia, with superimposed muscle twitches. REM sleep thus consists of tonic components (e.g., activated EEG, muscle atonia, suppression of reflexes) and phasic components (e.g., rapid eye movements, muscle twitches). About 20% to 25% of the night is spent in REM sleep.

REM sleep is sometimes referred to as "dreaming sleep," since dreaming is most common in this stage. Dreams are hallucinatory phenomena that are predominantly visual, although other sensory experiences, including auditory, tactile, and kinesthetic, may occur. The most common emotions in dreams are fear and anxiety. Dreams may be mundane or bizarre, but they differ from waking consciousness in that they are characterized by confusion, disorientation, and discontinuity (i.e., events are not logically connected). Although dreams are more frequent in REM sleep, they may also occur in NREM sleep, particularly lighter stages (N1 and N2). NREM dreams are generally shorter in duration and may be less bizarre than those occurring in REM sleep.

Monitoring human sleep, or **polysomnography**, consists of recording EEG, EOG, and chin EMG to define the stages of sleep and waking, as well as other physiological parameters. Characteristic EEG waveforms of various sleep stages and waking are prominent over different parts of the brain, so EEG electrodes are applied over frontal (to measure slow waves), central (for sleep spindles), and occipital regions (for alpha activity) to better distinguish stages of sleep and wakefulness. A sleep study or **polysomnogram** will typically also include recording of nasal/oral airflow, respiratory effort, snoring, electrocardiogram, oxyhemoglobin saturation, limb EMG, body position, and video recording to document behaviors during sleep; other parameters may be recorded depending on the clinical symptoms.

How Much Sleep Do We Need?

Human sleep need varies by age and among individuals; the amount of sleep needed is that which results in no daytime sleepiness or dysfunction. Most adults report obtaining about 7 hours of sleep per night. Epidemiological studies suggest that about 7 to 8 hours of sleep per night is optimal for

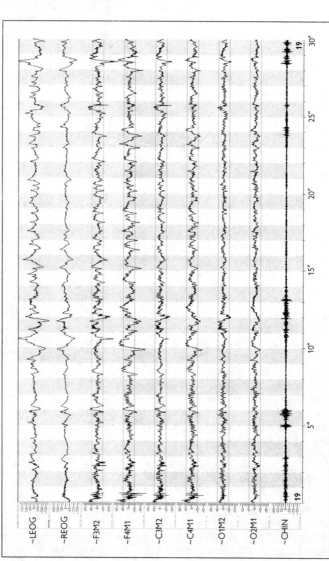

Figure 1.1 Waking with eyes open. Note the frequent, irregular eye movements in the EOG channels (subject watching TV). LEOG, Left electrooculogram; REOG, Right electrooculogram; F3M2, F4M1, Frontal EEG channels; C3M2, C4M1, Central EEG channels; Chin, Chin electromyogram.

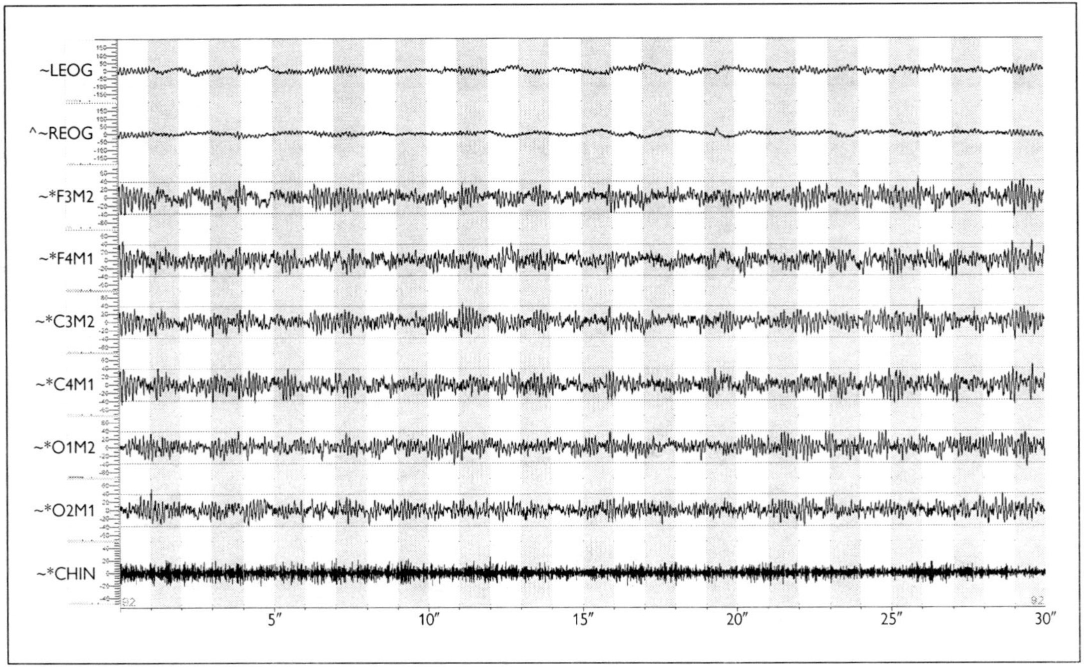

Figure 1.2 Waking with eyes closed. Note prominent alpha rhythm in EEG. LEOG, Left electro-oculogram; REOG, Right electrooculogram; F3M2, F4M1, Frontal EEG channels; C3M2, C4M1, Central EEG channels; Chin, Chin electromyogram.

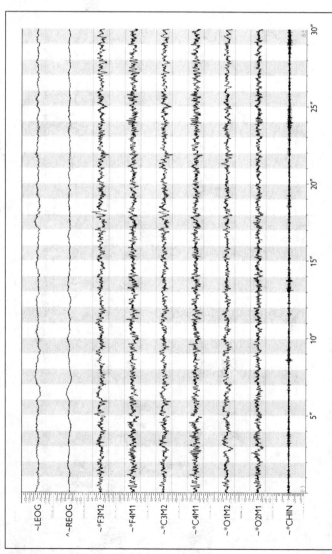

Figure 1.3 Stage N1. LEOG, Left electrooculogram; REOG, Right electrooculogram; F3M2, F4M1, Frontal EEG channels; C3M2, C4M1, Central EEG channels; Chin, Chin electromyogram.

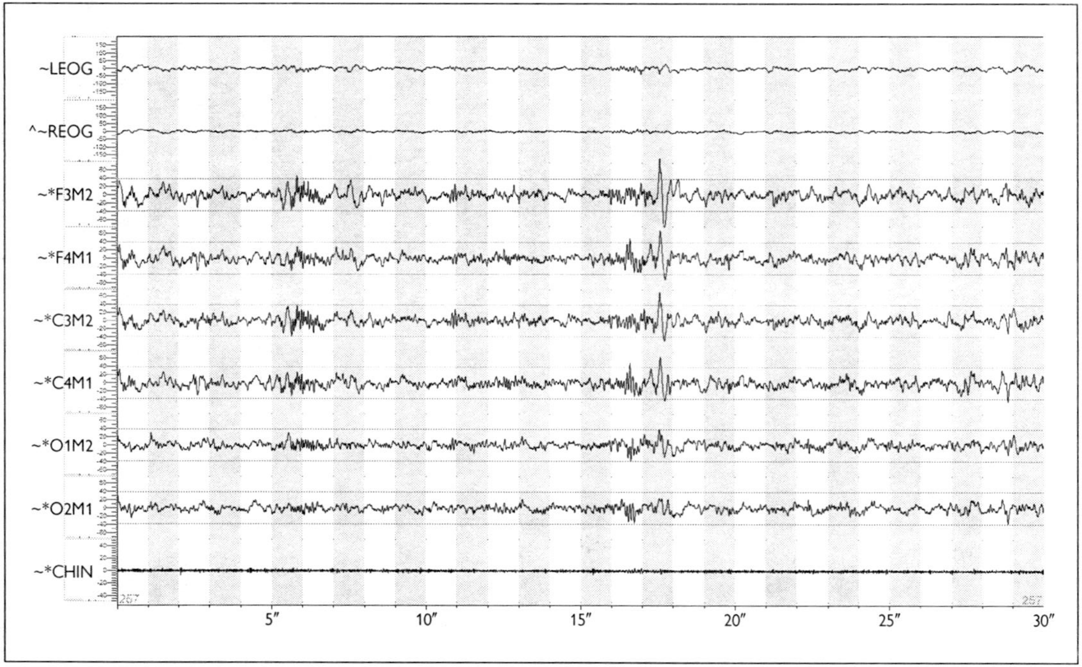

Figure 1.4 Stage N2. Note sleep spindles and vertex sharp waves in EEG. LEOG, Left electrooculogram; REOG, Right electrooculogram; F3M2, F4M1, Frontal EEG channels; C3M2, C4M1, Central EEG channels; Chin, Chin electromyogram.

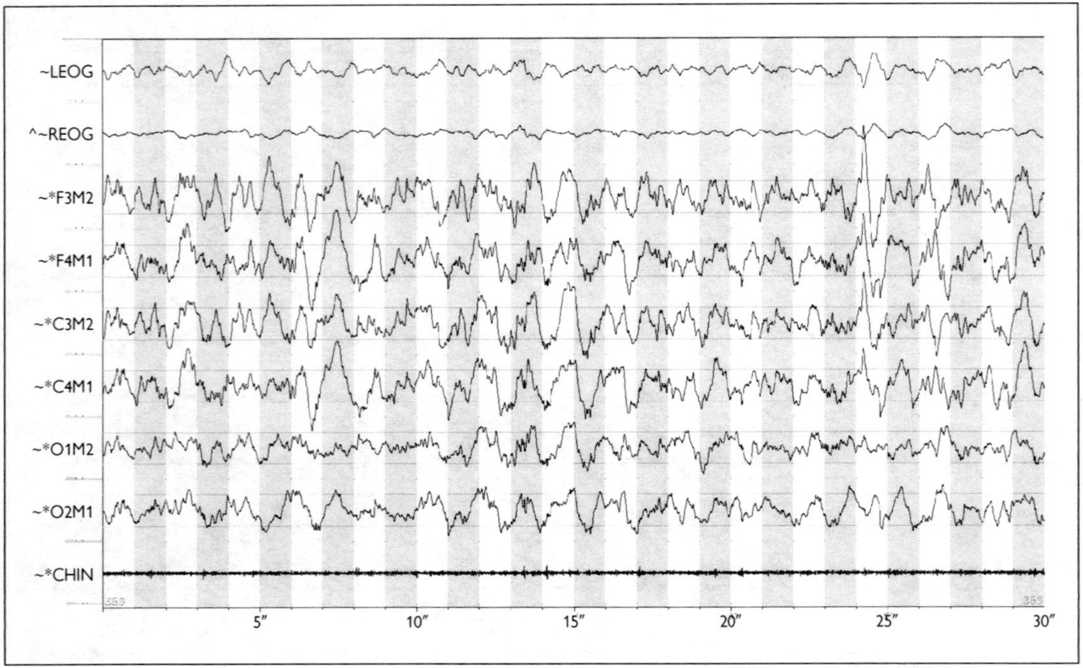

Figure 1.5 Stage N3. Note prominent slow waves in EEG. LEOG, Left electrooculogram; REOG, Right electrooculogram; F3M2, F4M1, Frontal EEG channels; C3M2, C4M1, Central EEG channels; Chin, Chin electromyogram.

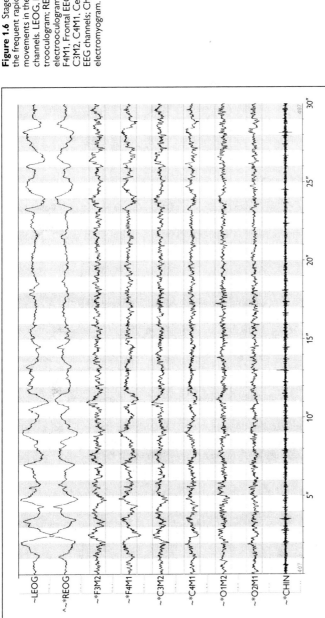

Figure 1.6 Stage R. Note the frequent rapid eye movements in the EOG channels. LEOG, Left electrooculogram; REOG, Right electrooculogram; F3M2, F4M1, Frontal EEG channels; C3M2, C4M1, Central EEG channels; Chin, Chin electromyogram.

health maintenance for the majority of individuals.[3] Some otherwise healthy individuals may be short sleepers (getting <6 hours per night without requiring "catch-up" sleep on weekends) or long sleepers (requiring 10 or more hours of sleep per night). Individuals who sleep shorter or longer than the norm have an increased mortality risk[4]; although sleep duration appears to be predictive of death in prospective studies, a causal link has not been established. Women typically sleep about 45 minutes longer than men per night.

How is Sleep Organized?

Regardless of the duration of the sleep period, sleep usually follows a typical pattern across the night in normal adults who go to bed and wake up at more or less the same times every day. The nocturnal sleep period consists of alternating periods of NREM and REM sleep; these NREM/REM sleep cycles each last about 90 minutes or more. Normally, sleep is initiated through NREM sleep, starting with a brief period of stage N1 sleep, followed by N2 and then N3. REM sleep typically follows a period of stage N2. Stage N3 amounts are usually greatest during the first cycle of NREM sleep, at the beginning of the night, and diminish or disappear later in the night. REM sleep bouts, on the other hand, are longer and dreaming is more intense during the later part of the night.

How Does Sleep Change Across the Lifespan?

Sleep begins during fetal life and differentiates into precursors of REM and NREM sleep by the third trimester. At birth, infants spend 16 to 18 hours per day sleeping, and they have short sleep–wake cycles of about 3 to 4 hours that are distributed across the day, without a clear day–night pattern. Up to 50% of sleep in newborns consists of REM sleep. Infants also enter sleep through REM sleep until about 3 to 4 months of age, when they switch to initiating sleep through NREM sleep. At this point, they also start to consolidate their sleep more during the night, and by 6 to 9 months of age most babies can sleep through the night. Daytime sleep consists of shorter naps as periods of wakefulness become more sustained. The most dramatic change during the first years of life is the reduction of total sleep, largely due to elimination or reduction of

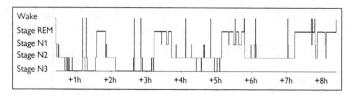

Figure 1.7 Hypnogram of a normal adult.

daytime napping. Sleep amount continues to decrease during childhood and adolescence.

There are also significant changes in sleep stages across development.[5] SWS (stage N3) is greatest in prepubertal children and clinically associated with a high arousal threshold. Not surprisingly, SWS parasomnias (e.g., confusional arousals, sleepwalking) are more prevalent in this age group. During adolescence, SWS and total sleep time decrease, and changes in the circadian clock lead teenagers to prefer to stay up later and sleep in later in the morning.

Age-related sleep changes during adulthood include a continuing decline in SWS and increasing fragmentation of sleep by brief arousals, leading to decreased efficiency of sleep across the night. SWS may be absent in older adults. Small declines in REM sleep amounts also occur with advanced age. Older adults tend to describe their sleep as "less deep" as a result of these changes, and insomnia complaints become more prevalent. Daytime sleepiness and napping increase as well. However, elderly individuals also have higher rates of medical and psychiatric illnesses as well as an increased prevalence of sleep disorders, which may contribute to their increased sleep complaints. Individuals with Alzheimer's disease and other causes of dementia show even more significant disruption of sleep organization; in severe cases, there may be almost complete loss of day–night organization of wakefulness and sleep and greater loss of REM sleep. Age-related changes in sleep are shown in Figure 1.8.

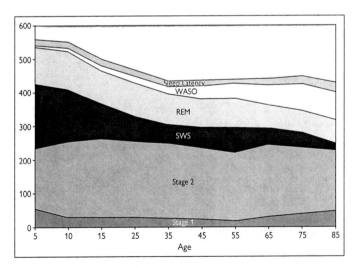

Figure 1.8 Age-related changes in sleep. Reproduced with permission: Ohayon MM, Carskadon MA, Guilleminault C, Vitiello MV. Meta-analysis of quantitative sleep parameters from childhood to old age in healthy individuals: developing normative sleep values across the human lifespan. WASO, wakefulness after sleep onset. *Sleep.* 2004;27(7):1255–1273. Copyright 2004 by American Academy of Sleep Medicine.

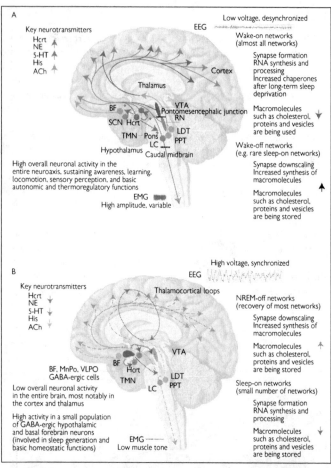

Figure 1.9 Activity of major neural networks and hypothesized molecular processes occurring during (A) wake, (B) NREM sleep, and (C) REM sleep. Neurotransmitter abbreviations: NE, norepinephrine; His, histamine; 5-HT, serotonin; Ach, acetylcholine; and Hcrt, hypocretin peptide. Anatomical abbreviations: BF, basal forebrain (Ach and GABA populations); LDT, laterodorsal tegmental cholinergic (Ach) nucleus; PPT, mesopontine pedunculopontine tegmental cholinergic (Ach) nucleus; LC, adrenergic (NE) locus coeruleus; RN, serotoninergic (5-HT) raphe nuclei; TMN, histaminergic (His) tuberomammillary nucleus; VTA, dopaminergic ventral tegmental area; mPO, median preoptic hypothalamic (GABA) systems; VLPO, ventrolateral preoptic hypothalamic (GABA) systems; SLC, sublocus coeruleus area (GABA and glutamatergic cell groups); SCN, suprachiasmatic nucleus; and Hcrt, hypocretin/orexin containing cell group. Upward and downward arrows represent increased/decreased activity and release for selected neurotransmitter (e.g., Ach, NE, 5-HT, His, and Hcrt) systems or in selected metabolic pathways (e.g., protein biosynthesis) during the corresponding sleep/wake state. Reprinted from Mignot E. Why we sleep: the temporal organization of recovery. *PLoS Biol.* Apr 29 2008;6(4):e106.

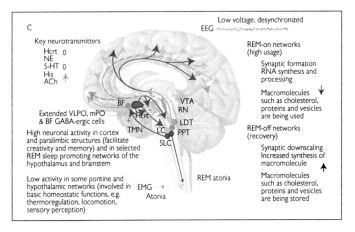

C

Low voltage, desynchronized
EEG

Key neurotransmitters
Hcrt 0
NE
5-HT 0
His
ACh

REM-on networks
(high usage)

Synaptic formation
RNA synthesis and
processing

Macromolecules
such as cholesterol,
proteins and vesicles
are being used

BF   VTA
                            RN

Extended VLPO, mPO   Hcrt
& BF GABA-ergic cells   LDT

High neuronal activity in cortex   TMN   LC PPT
and paralimbic structures (facilitate   SLC
creativity and memory) and in selected
REM sleep promoting networks of the
hypothalamus and brainstem

REM-off networks
(recovery)

Synaptic downscaling
Increased synthesis of
macromolecule

Low activity in some pontine and   REM atonia
hypothalamic networks (involved in   EMG
basic homeostatic functions, e.g.   Atonia
thermoregulation, locomotion,
sensory perception)

Macromolecules
such as cholesterol,
proteins and vesicles
are being stored

Figure 1.9 Continued.

How is Sleep Regulated?

States of sleep and wakefulness are regulated by multiple and interacting brain systems. Sleep is not merely the absence of wakefulness but an active process, with different mechanisms for NREM and REM stages. Wakefulness and sleep states are each reinforced by multiple systems, such that no single brain lesion can permanently eliminate sleep or waking; such mechanistic redundancy is necessary given the importance of these behaviors for survival.

Brain Systems Involved in Sleep and Wakefulness[6–8]

Wakefulness is primarily maintained by the ascending reticular activating system (ARAS), with two major components: (1) the dorsal tegmental or reticulothalamocortical pathway, which causes activation of the cortical EEG, and (2) the ventral tegmental or extrathalamic pathway, which produces arousal and waking behavior.

The dorsal tegmental pathway consists of projections from cholinergic neurons from the pedunculopontine (PPT) and laterodorsal tegmental (LDT) nuclei in the mesopontine tegmentum to the thalamus. This excitatory input in turn increases excitatory transmission from the thalamus to the cortex and produces cortical activation. Activity of PPT and LDT neurons is greatest during waking and REM sleep, states that are characterized by an activated EEG pattern. There are also direct cholinergic projections from cholinergic neurons in the basal forebrain to the cortex that increase firing rates during waking and REM sleep and contribute to cortical activation.

The ventral tegmental pathway comprises inputs from various monoaminergic nuclei that project to the hypothalamus, basal forebrain, and cerebral cortex; they include noradrenergic projections from the locus coeruleus (LC) in the rostral pons, dopaminergic projections from the ventral periaqueductal gray matter and ventral tegmental area, histaminergic projections from the tuberomammillary nucleus (TMN), and serotonergic projections from the dorsal raphe and median raphe nuclei. Firing rates of these noradrenergic, histaminergic, serotonergic, and possibly dopaminergic neurons are highest during waking, decreased in NREM sleep, and lowest or inactive during REM sleep.

One of the most important components of the ARAS is the glutamatergic input from the midbrain reticular formation; glutamate is the major excitatory neurotransmitter in the brain. The reticular formation is active during waking and REM sleep and contributes to both arousal pathways with projections to the thalamus, basal forebrain, hypothalamus, and cerebral cortex. The reticular formation is activated by inputs from sensory and motor systems and thus is important for arousal in response to external or environmental stimulation.

Neurons that secrete hypocretin (also called orexin), found in the perifornical region of the lateral and posterior hypothalamus, serve to reinforce arousal by sending excitatory projections back to the various nuclei in the ARAS, particularly the LC, as well as widespread projections to the cerebral cortex. The hypocretin system appears to be particularly important for stabilizing behavioral state; the disorder narcolepsy, characterized by frequent sleep attacks during wakefulness as well as fragmentation of nocturnal sleep, has been associated with unusually low levels of hypocretin in the cerebrospinal fluid.

Medications that act on these neurotransmitter systems thus can have significant effects on arousal levels. Those with cholinergic effects promote cortical arousal; anticholinergic medications decrease arousal levels or promote sedation. Amphetamines produce arousal by increasing levels of dopamine and norepinephrine. Some antidepressants, including selective serotonin reuptake inhibitors (e.g., fluoxetine, sertraline) and combined serotonin and norepinephrine reuptake inhibitors (e.g., venlafaxine, duloxetine), as well as agents that are selective norepinephrine reuptake inhibitors (e.g., atomoxetine, used for Attention Deficit Hyperactivity Disorder), can also increase arousal levels in some individuals and/or contribute to insomnia. Antihistamines that act as antagonists to central histamine type 1 or 2 (H1 or H2) receptors, on the other hand, can produce sedation.

NREM sleep is thought to be initiated through activation of groups of neurons in the anterior hypothalamus and basal forebrain, including the ventrolateral preoptic nucleus (VLPO) and median preoptic nucleus. These neurons are preferentially active during sleep and release the inhibitory neurotransmitters gamma-amino butyric acid (GABA) and galanin; GABA is the major inhibitory neurotransmitter in the brain, and medications that increase GABA transmission, such as most hypnotics, increase NREM sleep amounts. The sleep-active cells project to the major arousal centers, including the LC, dorsal and median raphe nuclei, and hypocretin neurons in the lateral hypothalamus. These arousal systems, in turn, project to and inhibit the sleep-initiating neurons, and it has been suggested that this reciprocal innervation functions much like an electrical "flip-flop" switch to promote state stability and avoid rapid shifts between sleep and waking, in that each system (sleep or waking) reinforces itself and inhibits the other state.[7]

One of the characteristics of NREM sleep is the deactivation of the cortical EEG and many brain structures. As excitatory glutamatergic and cholinergic input to the thalamus decreases, thalamocortical cells are inhibited and sensory stimuli are mostly prevented from reaching the cortex. This disfacilitation leads to the expression of intrinsic rhythms in thalamocortical cells in the reticular nucleus of the thalamus and the appearance of sleep spindles and K-complexes in the EEG. As hyperpolarization of the thalamus increases, slow oscillations generated in the thalamocortical and cortical neurons appear and give rise to slow waves (delta waves), characteristic of SWS. Another important component of NREM sleep is the sleep-promoting effect of adenosine transmission in the basal forebrain. Adenosine is a degradation product of ATP; its levels build up in the basal forebrain during wakefulness and decrease during sleep. It is likely that increased adenosine levels are responsible for contributing to the homeostatic drive for sleep that results from prolonged wakefulness. Caffeine, the most commonly used substance to promote waking, acts by antagonizing adenosine receptors.

A multitude of other substances have also been shown to contribute to promotion of NREM sleep, including interleukin 1, tumor necrosis factor, prostaglandin D2, and nitric oxide.[9] These compounds are all increased during inflammation and may account for the increased sleepiness that occurs in many illnesses, particularly infectious ones.

The critical structures for the initiation of **REM sleep** are groups of cholinergic and cholinoceptive neurons in the pons and caudal midbrain, including the LDT and PPT regions; these structures are necessary and sufficient to generate REM sleep. Medications that have cholinergic effects (e.g., reserpine) can increase REM sleep, whereas anticholinergic agents reduce REM sleep amounts. As in waking, activation of the EEG is mediated by cholinergic projections to the thalamus. Muscle atonia is mediated by inhibitory input from the subceruleus area of the pons, below the LC, to neurons in the medullary reticular formation, which in turn inhibit spinal motor neurons through release of GABA and glycine. Destruction of the subceruleus area in animals can lead to REM sleep without atonia, similar to REM behavior disorder in humans.

Ponto-geniculo-occipital (PGO) waves are characteristic of REM sleep, although they are not typically seen on the EEG recorded from scalp electrodes. They are also associated with other aspects of brain function, including startle responses and cognitive functions. PGO waves are associated with phasic events in REM sleep, such as eye movements and muscle twitches, and originate from the subceruleus region. PGO-generating cells from the subceruleus input to a variety of areas; for example, projections to vestibular neurons activate oculomotor neurons to produce eye movements. They also project to many other structures, including the occipital cortex, amygdala, hippocampus, hypothalamus, pons, and medulla; these connections suggest that PGO waves may be important for initiating REM sleep as well as regulating REM sleep-dependent learning and memory.[10]

REM sleep is also regulated by interactions with aminergic cells; the LC and raphe nuclei inhibit the cholinergic/cholinoceptive REM sleep-initiating cells. The generation of REM sleep also appears to be influenced by the extended VLPO region, through GABAergic projections that inhibit these brainstem aminergic nuclei, thus allowing REM sleep to occur. The forebrain also appears to modulate REM sleep in that the amygdala and brain-stem REM-generating sites innervate each other and electrical stimulation or pharmacological stimulation of the amygdala can alter REM sleep expression[11]; this suggests that the amygdala may have an influence on the emotional aspects of dreaming.

Medications that increase cholinergic activity (e.g., agents used to treat Alzheimer's disease) tend to increase REM sleep amounts, whereas anticholinergic drugs suppress REM sleep. Agents that increase noradrenergic or serotonergic activity, such as most antidepressants, also tend to suppress REM sleep through aminergic inhibition of the REM sleep-generating neurons.

Circadian and Homeostatic Regulation of Sleep[12–15]

The overall organization of sleep and wakefulness across the day is organized by two processes: the homeostatic drive for sleep and the circadian rhythm. The two-process model developed by Alexander Borbely explains sleep propensity as an interaction between these two processes (Fig. 1.10).[12] The homeostatic drive for sleep, process S, increases with prolonged wakefulness across the day and diminishes with sleep during the night. The circadian rhythm for sleep and alertness, process C, is such that sleep propensity is greatest in the early morning hours, during the latter part of the sleep period, and wakefulness is maximal in the early evening, several hours before sleep onset. Sleep onset at night is due to the buildup of process S, which is also associated with the predominance of SWS in the beginning of the sleep period. As discussed above, the mechanism for process S may include buildup of adenosine in the basal forebrain.

As the night progresses, process S diminishes but the circadian sleep tendency is increasing, allowing sleep to continue during the latter part of the night. It is not unusual for a period of wakefulness to occur during the night, as the homeostatic drive to sleep (process S) diminishes and before the circadian drive to sleep (process C) is maximal. REM sleep propensity is strongly linked to process C, so that REM sleep amounts are greatest during the later part of the night.

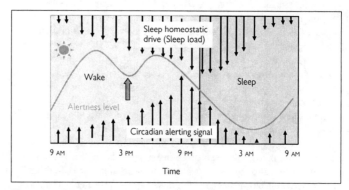

Figure 1.10 Schematic representation of the two-process model of sleep regulation. The homeostatic process increases during waking and decreases during sleep. The circadian process is independent of sleep and waking and interacts with the homeostatic process. Adapted from the American Academy of Sleep Medicine.

Conversely, upon waking up in the morning, the circadian alerting signal is relatively low. Arousal occurs because the homeostatic drive to sleep has been satiated, although other factors such as increased activity in the hypothalamic-pituitary-adrenal (HPA) axis also contribute to arousal (see below). As the day progresses, the homeostatic drive to sleep begins to build and the circadian alerting signal starts to increase but has not peaked; this leads to a period of increased sleep tendency in the afternoon, which generally improves later in the day as the circadian alerting tendency increases further. Individuals who are somewhat sleep-deprived due to sleep disorders or insufficient sleep, or who are taking sedating medications, may have more difficulty staying awake through this period. In many cultures, people take naps or siestas at this time.

Circadian rhythms are found in every life form on earth. They are endogenously generated biological rhythms that have a period of about 24 hours; they are not simply passive responses to the light–dark cycle in that they can persist even in the absence of time cues. In humans, circadian rhythms are generated from the primary circadian pacemaker in the suprachiasmatic nucleus (SCN) of the hypothalamus. The SCN regulates various physiological functions and behaviors to organize physiology and behavior across the day. Examples of circadian outputs include sleep–wakefulness, core body temperature, neuroendocrine function, and renal function.

Circadian rhythms are entrained to the 24-hour day by a variety of cues or zeitgebers ("time givers"). The most important and potent zeitgeber is light, but other factors such as feeding schedules, physical activity, and social interactions can also affect the relationship between the endogenous circadian rhythm and the environment. Inputs from various brain regions to the SCN mediate these entraining influences, most notably the retinohypothalamic tract for light input. Melatonin secretion by the pineal at night also serves to reinforce circadian entrainment.

Aspects of the circadian clock such as the endogenous period are genetically determined, and individuals with unusually short or long periods may be more likely to develop circadian rhythm sleep disorders. Problems with entrainment can also lead to sleep problems, whether related to changes in the sleep schedule such as in shift workers, or in adolescents who habitually stay up late at night.

What are the Effects of Sleep on Physiological Systems?

Both NREM and REM sleep are associated with significant changes in physiology. Sleep may thus have significant effects on a variety of medical disorders, and sleep disorders may have an impact on normal physiological processes and medical and psychiatric disorders.

Autonomic Nervous System

During NREM sleep, autonomic nervous system activity becomes more stable, with the greatest stability during SWS. Sympathetic activity remains at or below levels in relaxed wakefulness, whereas parasympathetic activity increases. During REM sleep, however, the autonomic nervous system becomes unstable, with brief surges in both sympathetic and parasympathetic activity that result in increased variability and extreme values for respiratory and cardiovascular parameters. Sympathetic surges accompany phasic REM events (eye movements, muscle twitches), whereas parasympathetic increases tend to occur during tonic REM sleep.

Cardiovascular System

As a result of increased autonomic nervous system stability in NREM sleep, heart rate, blood pressure, and cardiac output decrease and become more regular; they reach their lowest mean values during SWS (stage N3). During REM sleep, bursts of sympathetic activity lead to transient increases in heart rate and blood pressure; increased parasympathetic activity causes heart rate decelerations. Individuals with heart disease are thus at greater risk for myocardial infarction or arrhythmias during REM sleep. They may also be at risk for cardiac events or stroke related to hypotension in NREM sleep.

Respiratory System

Regulation of the respiratory system during sleep is affected not only by changes in autonomic control, but also by sleep-related changes in chemical and mechanical control of breathing. There is also an increased ventilatory drive during wakefulness that disappears during sleep. During NREM sleep, the ventilatory responses to hypoxia and hypercapnia are reduced compared to wakefulness and decrease even further during REM sleep. As a result of these changes, periodic breathing may be seen transiently at sleep onset, particularly in individuals with greater hypercapnic ventilatory responses. The Cheyne-Stokes respiration that develops in heart failure patients is characterized by increased ventilation in response to hypercarbia, followed by an apneic response until the partial pressure of CO_2 falls below the threshold for ventilation.

Sleep is also accompanied by increased resistance to airflow, primarily in the upper airway. Relaxation of upper airway muscles occurs during sleep and can contribute to snoring and sleep apnea in susceptible individuals. The intercostal muscles (accessory respiratory muscles) become hypotonic in NREM sleep and atonic in REM sleep. These mechanical changes are associated with decreases in tidal volume and minute ventilation.

Overall, the reduced ventilatory drive, changes in chemical control of ventilation, and increased airway resistance during sleep can lead to increased respiratory compromise in patients with obstructive or restrictive lung disease, as well as those with heart failure or cardiac disease. They also contribute to the development of sleep-related breathing disorders (see Chapter 4).

Temperature Regulation

Temperature regulation during sleep is affected both by the circadian rhythm as well as by sleep itself. The circadian pattern of core body temperature is maximal in the early evening, several hours before sleep onset, and drops to its minimum in the early morning, several hours before waking up. Separate from circadian regulation of temperature, NREM sleep, particularly SWS, decreases the hypothalamic temperature set point and leads to active heat loss (cutaneous vasodilation and sweating). These two factors lead to the experience of going to bed feeling somewhat cold, and waking up feeling too warm and sweaty several hours later. During REM sleep, thermoregulatory mechanisms such as sweating and shivering are significantly reduced, leading to a decreased ability to regulate body temperature during this state.

Environmental temperature, in turn, can have profound effects on sleep. Excessively cold or warm temperatures cause frequent arousals and decreases in both REM and NREM sleep amounts. Passive body heating several hours prior to sleep, however, can increase SWS and has been used to improve sleep in patients with insomnia.

Endocrine System

Many hormones are regulated by the circadian system and also show variation in response to sleep and wakefulness. Hormones whose secretion is particularly related to sleep and wakefulness are growth hormone (GH) and prolactin (PRL). A pulse of GH secretion occurs shortly after sleep onset, stimulated by SWS. GH, in turn, seems to increase SWS amounts. In individuals with fragmented sleep, GH levels can be significantly reduced. PRL release also increases during sleep, with greatest release during the middle of the sleep period.

Thyroid-stimulating hormone (TSH) is under circadian control; TSH release peaks in the evening prior to sleep onset and is further stimulated by sleep deprivation. Sleep onset suppresses TSH release at night, but naps during the day do not seem to interfere with TSH levels.

Activity of the HPA axis shows a circadian pattern of increased adrenocorticotropic hormone (ACTH) and cortisol release in the morning, beginning prior to awakening and peaking in the early morning; increased activity of the HPA axis appears to contribute to awakening in the morning. HPA axis activity decreases across the day, reaching a minimum in the evening and during the beginning of the nocturnal sleep period. SWS also inhibits cortisol secretion during the first part of the night.

Melatonin is regulated by the circadian system and the light–dark cycle. In terms of its circadian pattern, it can be released only during the night, but its secretion is suppressed by bright light. As a result, the onset of melatonin secretion is earlier and the offset is later in the winter, when the period of daylight is shorter. The duration of melatonin release across the night thus provides a signal regarding day length and is involved in the regulation of seasonal breeding patterns in many mammals. It also has feedback effects on the circadian clock (see below) and may have some sleep-promoting effects; melatonin and melatonin agonists are increasingly used to treat a variety of sleep disorders.

Reproductive System

REM sleep is associated with penile erections that begin in infancy and continue into old age. Organic causes of impotence may often be distinguished from psychological causes through measurement of sleep-related changes in penile tumescence. Women experience clitoral erections and increased vaginal blood flow during REM sleep. Although penile and clitoral erections occur in REM sleep, they are not necessarily associated with sexual dream content.

What are the Effects of Insufficient Sleep?

The primary effect of sleep deprivation or insufficient sleep is sleepiness. After extended sleep loss, a "sleep rebound" usually occurs, meaning that the individual obtains more sleep than usual for the night and/or sleep may be more intense, with increased N3 and slow-wave activity. Latency to sleep onset is shorter than usual, and sleep efficiency is usually increased. With prolonged sleep deprivation, REM sleep rebound may also occur.

Sleep deprivation leads to cognitive impairment due to increased sleepiness and state instability, as well as to effects on brain systems involved in attention and cognition.[16,17] Sleep loss leads to decreased activity in brain regions involved in vigilance during cognitive tasks as well as to the occurrence of very brief episodes of stage N1 or N2 sleep, or "microsleeps." There is a general slowing of reaction time, which increases with longer duration of sleep loss that can lead to lapses in responding to stimuli. Prolonged lapses in attention occur as a result of microsleeps; severely sleep-deprived individuals can experience microsleeps despite their best efforts to try to remain awake. Attentional lapses are more likely to occur in situations that are boring or less stimulating, and also increase with longer time spent on the task; overall these changes are associated with decreased motivation. Attentional lapses can lead to accidents or injuries; a lapse or microsleep of only a few seconds can be sufficient to lead to a fatal traffic accident, for example. In fact, drowsy drivers show impairment comparable to drunk drivers. Sleep-deprived individuals also make errors of commission (i.e., responses in the absence of a stimulus); these "false alarms" can also lead to serious consequences.

Sleep deprivation not only impairs attention and arousal level, but it also has effects on a broad range of higher cognitive functions.[18] Significant decrements occur in cognitive throughput, mood, creative thinking, memory, logical reasoning, and ability to focus on multiple tasks simultaneously. Sleep loss also leads to errors in judgment and increases in risk-taking behavior. Sleep-deprived individuals typically underestimate their level of impairment, which further contributes to accidents and injuries.

Decrements in attention and cognition can occur with even a few hours of sleep loss, as well as with partial sleep deprivation. Chronic, daily sleep restriction occurs commonly in individuals who do not schedule sufficient time for sleep, as well as in those with sleep disorders that fragment sleep at night, such as sleep apnea. Individuals who obtain 6 or less hours of sleep per day show increased daytime sleepiness and decrements in psychomotor and cognitive tasks that progressively worsen with longer periods of sleep restriction.

There are also significant individual differences in responses to sleep deprivation that are related to genetic factors; some individuals can become severely impaired with relatively little sleep loss, whereas others function reasonably well despite fairly prolonged periods of sleep deprivation. These differences appear to be stable within individuals but can vary related to the nature of the task; individuals may show relatively preserved function on some types of tasks but impairment on others, and these patterns vary from person to person. No one, however, can go without sleep indefinitely, and individuals cannot "train" themselves to need less sleep by chronic sleep restriction.

Epidemiological studies have suggested that individuals living in industrialized societies such as the United States have significantly reduced their sleep time, and that chronic sleep loss leads to increased morbidity and mortality, including an increased risk for hypertension, diabetes, and cardiovascular disease.[3,17] Shorter sleep duration has been associated with increased BMI and an increased risk for obesity in children and adults in some studies.[19] These health outcomes may be related to the physiological effects of sleep loss, including increased sympathetic nervous system activation and effects on neuroendocrine and immune function. For example, shorter sleep duration has been associated with decreased glucose tolerance, increased cortisol levels, elevated blood pressure, increased inflammation, changes in immune function, and decreased serum levels of leptin and elevated levels of ghrelin, a hormone profile that can produce increased appetite.

What is the Function of Sleep?

Although much is known about the effects of sleep loss, the functions of sleep remain largely a mystery. Many theories have been proposed to explain why we need to spend such a large part of our lives in a state that appears to have otherwise little survival value and, in fact, puts us in a position of increased vulnerability by disconnecting us from the environment. Specific theories of sleep have addressed functions of NREM and REM sleep separately, since the two states are so biologically distinct and thus may have different purposes. NREM sleep may help to replenish substances or factors that are expended during wakefulness, such as glycogen, proteins, or energy stores, although the data in support of these ideas are not strong. No single hypothesis appears sufficient to explain sleep, and it is likely that sleep subserves a number of critical functions.[6,20] Prolonged sleep deprivation in rats, including total sleep deprivation or selective REM sleep deprivation, invariably leads to death, suggesting that sleep is necessary for survival in at least some species.[21]

One group of hypotheses suggests that sleep is an adaptive behavioral response: a sleeping animal is out of harm's way during the period of the day that it does not need to be actively engaged in other activities and thus decreases the risk of predation. Another approach focuses on sleep as conserving energy by enforcing relative immobility. However, metabolic rate is only slightly reduced in sleep in comparison to quiet wakefulness, which does not justify the need for a prolonged period of decreased environmental awareness. Sleep thus appears to be primarily important for brain function, since there is no evidence that any other parts of the body require sleep rather than simply the rest that can be achieved through quiet wakefulness.

It has been proposed that SWS sleep serves to promote synaptic homeostasis in the brain.[22] During waking, brain activity related to learning produces long-term potentiation at synapses, leading to increased synaptic strength and resultant increases in energy and space requirements. With prolonged wakefulness, our capacity to learn is eventually compromised due to saturation of this process. However, sleep, through the occurrence of slow waves and other mechanisms, produces a generalized downscaling of these synapses back to a baseline level. This process of sleep-related synaptic homeostasis promotes learning and memory; sleep is thus required for brain plasticity. Another not mutually exclusive hypothesis has proposed that SWS may be associated with neural reactivation and thus synaptic potentiation of specific experience-dependent circuits, thus leading to memory improvement during sleep.[23] Sleep spindles, another key component of NREM sleep, have also been associated with sleep-dependent learning in some studies.

It has been suggested that REM sleep, on the other hand, may be important for the endogenous stimulation of important brain circuits such as those involved in the visual system and instinctual behaviors, or for periodic activation of the brain during sleep after periods of NREM sleep. REM sleep may also be important for emotional memory processing,[23] which may account for the association of mood disorders with abnormalities in REM sleep expression. The loss of REM sleep that may occur in individuals who are taking monoamine oxidase inhibitors for depression or who have certain brain lesions does not lead to obvious cognitive or emotional impairment in adults, however.

It is likely that the functions of sleep include aspects of a number of these theories. From a clinical standpoint, sleep is clearly important for brain development and optimal brain function and also has a significant impact on various physiological systems. It is therefore not surprising that impaired or inadequate sleep is associated with an increased risk for medical and psychiatric disorders, accidents, and injuries; decreased productivity; poorer quality of life; and increased all-cause mortality.

References

1. Rechtschaffen A, Kales A. *A Manual of Standardized Terminology, Techniques, and Scoring System for Sleep Stages of Human Subjects*. UCLA, Los Angeles: Brain Information Service/Brain Research Institute, 1968.

2. American Academy of Sleep Medicine. *The AASM Manual for the Scoring of Sleep and Associated Events: Rules, Terminology and Technical Specification*. Westchester, IL: American Academy of Sleep Medicine, 2007.

3. Bixler E. Sleep and society: an epidemiological perspective. *Sleep Med.* 2009 Sep;10 Suppl 1:S3–6.

4. Cappuccio FP, D'Elia L, Strazzullo P, Miller MA. Sleep duration and all-cause mortality: a systematic review and meta-analysis of prospective studies. *Sleep.* 2010 May 1;33(5):585–592.

5. Ohayon MM, Carskadon MA, Guilleminault C, Vitiello MV. Meta-analysis of quantitative sleep parameters from childhood to old age in healthy individuals: developing normative sleep values across the human lifespan. *Sleep.* 2004;27(7):1255–1273.

6. Mignot E. Why we sleep: the temporal organization of recovery. *PLoS Biol.* 2008 Apr 29;6(4):e106.

7. Fuller PM, Gooley JJ, Saper CB. Neurobiology of the sleep-wake cycle: sleep architecture, circadian regulation, and regulatory feedback. *J Biol Rhythms.* 2006 Dec;21(6):482–493.

8. Fort P, Bassetti CL, Luppi PH. Alternating vigilance states: new insights regarding neuronal networks and mechanisms. *Eur J Neurosci.* 2009 May;29(9):1741–1753.

9. Obal F, Jr., Krueger JM. Biochemical regulation of non-rapid-eye-movement sleep. *Front Biosci.* 2003 May 1;8:d520–550.

10. Datta S, Siwek DF, Patterson EH, Cipolloni PB. Localization of pontine PGO wave generation sites and their anatomical projections in the rat. *Synapse.* 1998 Dec;30(4):409–423.

11. Morrison AR, Sanford LD, Ross RJ. The amygdala: a critical modulator of sensory influence on sleep. *Biol Signals Recept.* 2000 Nov-Dec;9(6):283–296.

12. Borbely AA. A two-process model of sleep regulation. *Human Neurobiol.* 1982;1:195–204.

13. Czeisler CA, Buxton OM, Singh Khalsa SB. The human circadian timing system and sleep-wake regulation. In: Kryger M, Roth T, Dement W, eds. *Principles and Practice of Sleep Medicine*, 4th ed. Philadelphia, PA: Elsevier Saunders. 2005:375–394.

14. Dijk DJ, Lockley SW. Integration of human sleep-wake regulation and circadian rhythmicity. *J Appl Physiol.* 2002;92(2):852–862.

15. Achermann P, Borbely AA. Mathematical models of sleep regulation. *Front Biosci.* 2003 May 1;8:s683–693.

16. Lim J, Dinges DF. Sleep deprivation and vigilant attention. *Ann N Y Acad Sci.* 2008;1129:305–322.

17. Banks S, Dinges DF. Behavioral and physiological consequences of sleep restriction. *J Clin Sleep Med.* 2007 Aug 15;3(5):519–528.

18. Balkin TJ, Rupp T, Picchioni D, Wesensten NJ. Sleep loss and sleepiness: current issues. *Chest.* 2008 Sep;134(3):653–660.

19. Marshall NS, Glozier N, Grunstein RR. Is sleep duration related to obesity? A critical review of the epidemiological evidence. *Sleep Med Rev.* 2008 Aug;12(4):289–298.

20. Cirelli C, Tononi G. Is sleep essential? *PLoS Biol.* 2008 Aug 26;6(8):e216.

21. Rechtschaffen A. Current perspectives on the function of sleep. *Perspect Biol Med.* 1998;41(3):359–390.

22. Tononi G, Cirelli C. Sleep function and synaptic homeostasis. *Sleep Med Rev.* 2006 Feb;10(1):49–62.

23. Walker MP. The role of sleep in cognition and emotion. *Ann N Y Acad Sci.* 2009 Mar;1156:168–197.

Chapter 2

Clinical Evaluation of Sleep Disorders

The second edition of the International Classification of Sleep Disorders (ICSD-2) organizes sleep disorders into categories based on the presenting complaint and/or etiology.[1] There are six major categories for sleep disorders that are covered in the subsequent chapters of this handbook: insomnia, sleep-related breathing disorders, excessive sleepiness and narcolepsy, circadian rhythm sleep disorders, parasomnias, and sleep-related movement disorders. In addition, there are two categories that cover isolated symptoms/normal variants and other disorders that do not seem to fit into another category; they are mentioned in this chapter and are included in other chapters where they are relevant or part of the differential diagnosis.

Given the high prevalence of sleep problems in the population, healthcare providers should ask all patients about sleep at every visit.[2] Careful attention to sleep should be given to individuals at greater risk for sleep disorders, including women, the elderly, and those with significant medical or psychiatric illnesses. Patients, even those with serious sleep problems, generally do not bring up issues related to their sleep with healthcare providers unless they are specifically asked.

Clinical Examination

Chief Complaint

The clinical evaluation of a patient with a possible sleep disorder begins with accurate identification of the sleep symptom(s), since this will direct the rest of the evaluation. Patients may have more than one complaint related to their sleep, and it is not unusual for a patient to have more than one sleep disorder (e.g., sleep apnea and restless legs). In addition to having the patient describe the sleep issues that are most troublesome, the clinician should screen patients for the following symptoms that will suggest categories of sleep disorders requiring further assessment or consideration.

Insomnia

- Does the patient have difficulty falling asleep or staying asleep, or does the patient awaken earlier than desired in the morning?
- What is the quality of the sleep obtained? Is it perceived as unrefreshing or nonrestorative?

- Potential disorders: Insomnia. Insomnia may also be present in other sleep disorders, including sleep-related breathing disorders and sleep-related movement disorders, for example.
- Is the patient unable to sleep at the desired schedule, but able to sleep on a self-selected schedule?
- Potential disorders: Circadian rhythm sleep disorders

Snoring or Breathing Difficulties During Sleep

- Does the patient snore at night, or wake up choking or gasping for air?
- Are pauses in breathing (apneas) observed by the bed partner or family members?
- Potential disorders: Sleep-related breathing disorders

Excessive Sleepiness

- Does the patient complain of sleeping for too many hours?
- Does the patient fall asleep easily in low-stimulus situations, such as sitting in a meeting, watching TV, riding in a car?
- Have there been any episodes of drowsy driving?
- Potential disorders: Sleep-related breathing disorders, hypersomnias

Restless Legs

- Does the patient have an urge to move his or her legs (often accompanied by uncomfortable, restless sensations) that occur while relaxing at night or in bed that are temporarily relieved by movement?
- Potential disorders: Sleep-related movement disorders

Unusual Behaviors During Sleep

- Does the patient have repetitive kicking or rhythmic movements before sleep onset or during sleep?
- Potential disorders: Sleep-related movement disorders
- Does the patient walk or engage in unusual behaviors during the night with little or no recollection the next day?
- Does the patient display violent or agitated behavior during sleep?
- Does the patient act out dreams?
- Does the patient have frequent nightmares?
- Does the patient have teeth grinding during sleep?
- Potential disorders: Parasomnias, nocturnal seizures

History

Once the chief sleep complaints have been identified, further questioning about specific symptoms should be based on the specific diagnoses under consideration. The sleep history should contain the following general elements, however:

1. For each symptom, when the symptom first began to occur and any relevant circumstances at that time (e.g., other illnesses, stressors, medication or substance use)
2. For each symptom, the frequency, severity, and time of occurrence during the day or night

3. Sleep pattern, including bedtime and wake-up time, regularity of sleep schedule (weekdays, weekends), time from lights-out to sleep onset, number and duration of awakenings during the night, cause of nocturnal awakenings if known (e.g., nocturia, pain), ease of falling back to sleep after nocturnal awakening, whether awakening in the morning is spontaneous or requires an alarm
4. Bedtime routine, including how soon prior to bedtime this is initiated. Does the patient watch TV or use a computer in the bedroom, and how soon prior to sleep onset is this terminated?
5. The patient's work schedule. Does the patient work nights, or have a work schedule that switches timing of shifts, or are there other significant schedule changes that occur?
6. Any sleep-disruptive factors that occur near bedtime, such as exercise, bright light exposure, or heavy meals
7. Sleep environment, including noise, temperature, light level, mattress comfort, disruption from bed partner (e.g., snoring), disruption from family members (e.g., children who waken frequently or other caretaking responsibilities), presence of pets in bedroom
8. Daytime napping, including frequency, time of day, duration
9. General pattern of daytime activities, including exercise (type, time of day, frequency, duration), regularity of daily schedule
10. Effects of sleep problems on daytime function, including sleepiness, fatigue, mood, anxiety, pain, etc.

Medical and Psychiatric History

Relevant medical and psychiatric disorders should be noted, including whether sleep problems may be secondary to undertreated or undiagnosed illnesses; these are discussed in the chapters related to specific disorders.

Medications

Medications, both prescription and over-the-counter, should be reviewed for possible effects on sleep or exacerbation of sleep disorders; these are discussed in the chapters related to specific disorders.

Substance Use

Use of alcohol, caffeine, and tobacco products should be documented. Alcohol is commonly used to help promote sleep, and although it may help induce sleep at the beginning of the night, it typically disrupts sleep during the latter part of the night. Chronic alcohol use/abuse can lead to insomnia and nonrestorative sleep. Caffeine is a stimulant; it should be used in moderation and avoided for at least 8 hours prior to sleep onset in those with insomnia. Nicotine is also a stimulant and should be avoided prior to bedtime. Individuals using nicotine patches for smoking cessation should consider removing them at night if insomnia is a problem.

Family History

Many sleep disorders have genetic components and tend to run in families, such as sleep apnea and restless legs and circadian rhythm disorders. Others, such as insomnia, may be influenced by behavioral as well as possible genetic factors within families.

Social History

Occupations that require night or rotating shift work, or frequent travel across time zones may lead to circadian rhythm disorders.

Physical Examination

Vital signs, including blood pressure, height, and weight, should be obtained on every patient, since obesity and hypertension are risk factors for sleep-related breathing disorders. Physical examination relevant to the sleep disorders in question should be performed (e.g., examination of upper airway, lungs, cardio-vascular system for suspected sleep apnea; neurological examination for sleep-related movement disorders). In addition, a general physical examination may uncover other medical problems that may be contributing to sleep disturbance. For instance, an increased neck circumference (>17 inches in men, >16 inches in women) is associated with an increased risk for sleep apnea.

Laboratory Testing

Laboratory testing is based on the medical and sleep disorders diagnoses under consideration (e.g., ferritin and iron panel for restless legs; thyroid functions for possible sleep apnea).

Sleep Log or Diary

It is always useful to have patients fill out a sleep diary or sleep log for at least 1 week as part of the diagnostic evaluation. Sleep log data are required for at least 1 week for the diagnosis of circadian rhythm sleep disorders, and such information is particularly helpful when assessing insomnias and hypersomnias. Sleep logs are also useful in monitoring treatment response. An example is provided in Appendix 6.

Sleep Questionnaires

A variety of standardized, brief, self-report questionnaires are available to assess sleep-related symptoms. They have been validated in clinical populations, and although they are not sufficient to make a diagnosis of a specific sleep disorder, they can identify individuals who may require further evaluation. They can also be used in follow-up to assess response to treatment.

1. Epworth Sleepiness Scale[3]: Measures propensity to fall asleep in low-stimulus situations; useful to identify problem sleepiness (see Appendix 5)
2. Insomnia Severity Index[4]: Measures severity of insomnia and is sensitive to treatment effects (see Appendix 7)
3. Fatigue Severity Scale[5]: Measures fatigue, which is seen in patients with a variety of chronic illnesses, depression, and sleep disorders
4. International Restless Legs Severity Scale[6]: Measures presence and severity of restless legs symptoms
5. Berlin Questionnaire for Sleep Apnea[7]: Identifies patients at risk for sleep apnea (see Appendix 4)
6. Morningness–Eveningness Questionnaire[8]: Determines an individual's tendency to be a morning type (phase-advanced circadian rhythm) or evening type (phase-delayed circadian rhythm) (see Appendix 9)

Other scales may be useful in certain patients with sleep disorders to screen for the presence of significant anxiety or depression; patients with elevated scores on these scales require further evaluation for the presence of mood or anxiety disorder.

1. Beck Depression Inventory[9]: Measures severity of depressive symptoms.
2. Center for Epidemiologic Studies Depression Scale (CES-D)[10]: Measures severity of depressive symptoms; elevated scores are also found in those with anxiety disorders (see Appendix 11)

Sleep Laboratory Evaluation

Based on the findings from the clinical examination, some patients may require evaluation in the sleep laboratory. Patients who might need sleep laboratory testing should generally be referred to a sleep specialist, who can determine what type of testing is indicated. In some cases, such as patients with clear-cut symptoms of apnea, patients may be referred directly for sleep testing first. An understanding of the types of sleep tests available and their indications is useful for providing appropriate clinical information for the referral process, setting patient expectations, and interpreting the clinical information provided by the tests.

Polysomnography (PSG)

Description
Overnight PSG refers to the recording of multiple physiological parameters during the night by a technician in a sleep laboratory. A clinical sleep study, or polysomnogram, should ideally record the following parameters:[11]

1. Electroencephalogram (EEG) recorded from standard frontal, central, and occipital sites on the scalp (International 10–20 system for EEG electrode placement): F4-M1, C4-M1, O2-M1; backup electrodes should be placed at F3-M2, C3-M2, O3-M2
2. Electro-oculogram (EOG) measured from electrodes placed around the eyes
3. Electromyogram (EMG) recorded from electrodes placed below the chin
4. Electrocardiogram (ECG) recorded from torso electrode, with ECG lead II display
5. Leg EMG measured with electrodes placed over the anterior tibialis muscles on each leg
6. Airflow parameters, usually measured with an oronasal thermal sensor and nasal pressure sensor
7. Respiratory effort parameters, usually measured with respiratory inductance plethysmography (measurement of chest and abdominal volume using external sensors) or esophageal manometry (gold standard but less commonly performed due to need to insert esophageal balloons or catheters)
8. Oxygen saturation measured with pulse oximetry

9. Body position
10. Snoring and vocalizations during sleep measured with microphone
11. Video recording of behavior

Ideally, the patient should be recorded for the duration of his or her typical sleep period. PSG may also include titration of positive airway pressure therapy and/or oxygen for patients with sleep-related breathing disorders, in which case these parameters are also recorded (see Chapter 4).

Indications

PSG is usually indicated for diagnosis of the following conditions or in the following situations:[12]

1. Sleep-related breathing disorders
2. Positive airway pressure titration in patients with sleep-related breathing disorders
3. To assess for obstructive sleep apnea (OSA) in patients about to undergo upper airway surgery for snoring or sleep apnea
4. As follow-up to document treatment efficacy in the following:
   a. Oral appliance therapy in patients with moderate to severe OSA
   b. Following surgical treatment for OSA
   c. If symptoms return after oral appliance therapy or surgical treatment of OSA
5. As follow-up in the following circumstances:
   a. After significant weight loss (at least 10% body weight) in a patient with a sleep-related breathing disorder receiving continuous positive airway pressure therapy
   b. After significant weight gain (at least 10% body weight) in a patient with a sleep-related breathing disorder receiving continuous positive airway pressure therapy, with increased symptoms
   c. In a patient with a sleep-related breathing disorders whose symptoms return after good initial response to continuous positive airway pressure therapy
6. In heart failure patients with symptoms of disturbed sleep, nocturnal dyspnea, or snoring, or if symptomatic despite optimal management of congestive heart failure
7. In patients with neuromuscular disorders and sleep-related symptoms
8. Narcolepsy (must be followed by multiple sleep latency test the following day)
9. Parasomnias with the following features:
   a. Unusual or atypical presentations
   b. Violent or potentially injurious to the patient or bed partner
   c. Cases with forensic considerations
   d. Cases that do not respond to conventional therapy
10. For possible sleep-related seizures when standard EEG and clinical evaluations are inconclusive; in these cases, extended bilateral EEG montage and video recordings should be used

11. Periodic limb movement disorder

PSG is *not* routinely indicated for the following conditions or situations:

1. Insomnia
2. Circadian rhythm sleep disorders
3. Chronic lung disease
4. Common, uncomplicated and non-injurious parasomnias
5. Patients with known seizure disorders without sleep-related complaints
6. Restless legs
7. Depression

Data Included in Report

PSG reports typically include the parameters listed below.[11] Rough guides to normative adult values for some variables are included in parentheses, although it is important to keep in mind that the "first-night effect" of sleeping in the laboratory and having multiple monitors attached can disrupt sleep in even normal individuals.

Sleep Scoring Data

1. Lights-out clock time
2. Lights-on clock time
3. Total sleep time; amount of time (hours and minutes) spent asleep from lights-out to lights-on
4. Total recording time; time from lights-out to lights-on (hours and minutes)
5. Sleep latency; time (minutes) from lights-out to first epoch of any stage of sleep (>5 minutes, 60 minutes)
7. Wake after sleep onset; time spent awake (minutes) in the period from sleep onset to lights-on
8. Percent sleep efficiency; total sleep time/total recording time × 100% (usually >85%; sleep efficiency >95% suggests sleep deprivation or increased sleep pressure)
9. Time in each stage (minutes)
10. Percent of total sleep time spent in each stage (age-related; see Chapter 1)

Arousal Events

1. Number of arousals; defined as shift in EEG frequency (including alpha, theta, or >16 Hz) lasting at least 3 seconds, following at least 10 seconds of stable sleep
2. Arousal index; number of arousals per hour of total sleep time

Respiratory Events

See Table 2.1 for respiratory event scoring and Figures 2.1 through 2.5 for examples.

1. Number of obstructive apneas
2. Number of mixed apneas
3. Number of central apneas
4. Number of hypopneas
5. Number of apneas + hypopneas

Table 2.1 Respiratory Events

Apnea

Airflow signal is decreased to <10% of baseline for at least 90% of the event.

Duration of event is at least 10 seconds.

Obstructive apnea is associated with continued or increased inspiratory effort.

Central apnea is associated with absent inspiratory effort.

Cheyne-Stokes breathing consists of waxing and waning pattern of respiratory effort and airflow.

Mixed apnea is associated with initial absence of inspiratory effort followed by resumed inspiratory effort during the latter part of the event.

Hypopnea

Airflow signal is decreased to <70% of baseline for at least 90% of the event.

Duration of event is at least 10 seconds.

There is an oxyhemoglobin desaturation of at least 4% associated with the event.

Respiratory effort-related arousal (RERA)

Increased respiratory effort or flattening of nasal pressure waveform lasting at least 10 seconds and leading to an arousal

Event does not meet criteria for apnea or hypopnea.

Adapted with permission from American Academy of Sleep Medicine. *The AASM Manual for the Scoring of Sleep and Associated Events: Rules, Terminology and Technical Specification.* Westchester, IL: American Academy of Sleep Medicine, 2007.

6. Apnea index; average number of apneas (all types combined) per hour of total sleep time

7. Hypopnea index; average number of hypopneas per hour of total sleep time

8. Apnea + hypopnea index (AHI); average number of apneas + hypopneas per hour of total sleep time (<5)

9. Number of respiratory effort-related arousals

10. Respiratory effort-related arousal index; average number of respiratory effort-related arousals per hour of total sleep time

11. Total number of oxygen desaturations ≥3% or ≥4%

12. Oxygen desaturation index; average number of oxygen desaturations ≥3% or ≥4% per hour of total sleep time

13. Continuous oxygen saturation, mean value

14. Minimum oxygen saturation during sleep

15. Occurrence of hypoventilation

16. Occurrence of Cheyne-Stokes breathing

Cardiac Events

1. Average heart rate during sleep

2. Highest heart rate during sleep

3. Highest heart rate during recording

4. Lowest heart rate observed during recording

5. Presence of the following:

    a. Bradycardia, asystole (report longest pause)

    b. Sinus tachycardia during sleep (report highest heart rate)

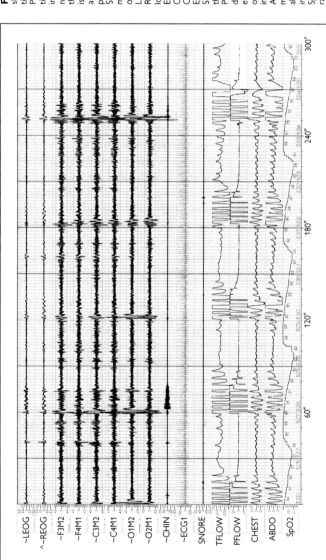

Figure 2.1 Obstructive sleep apneas. Note the cessation of flow in the Tflow and Pflow channels, but the continuation of respiratory effort in the Chest and Abdo channels. Initiation of breathing at the termination of each apnea is accompanied by arousal, as indicated by increased amplitude in the EEG channels. Significant drops in oxyhemoglobin saturation (SpO2) occur with apneas. LEOG, Left electrooculogram; REOG, Right electrooculogram; F3M2, F4M1, Frontal EEG channels; C3M2, C4M1, Central EEG channels; Chin, Chin electromyogram; ECG, Electrocardiogram; Snore, Snoring; Tflow, Oral-nasal thermistor measuring airflow; Pflow, Nasal pressure transducer; Chest, Respiratory effort measured at the level of the chest using respiratory inductance plethysmography; Abdo, Respiratory effort measured at the level of the abdomen using respiratory inductance plethysmography; SpO2, Percent oxygen saturation measured with pulse oximetry.

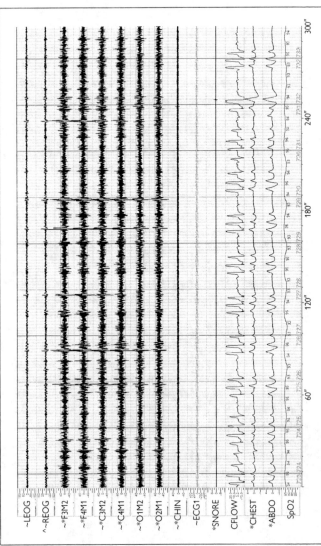

Figure 2.2 Central apneas (periodic breathing). Note the repetitive cessation in airflow (Tflow and Pflow channels) and respiratory effort (Chest and Abdo channels). Drops in oxyhemoglobin saturation (SpO2) occur with apneas. LEOG, Left electrooculogram; REOG, Right electrooculogram; F3M2, F4M1, Frontal EEG channels; C3M2, C4M1, Central EEG channels; Chin, Chin electromyogram; ECG, Electrocardiogram; Snore, Snoring; Tflow, Oral-nasal thermistor measuring airflow; Pflow, Nasal pressure transducer; Chest, Respiratory effort measured at the level of the chest using respiratory inductance plethysmography; Abdo, Respiratory effort measured at the level of the abdomen using respiratory inductance plethysmography; SpO2, Percent oxygen saturation measured with pulse oximetry.

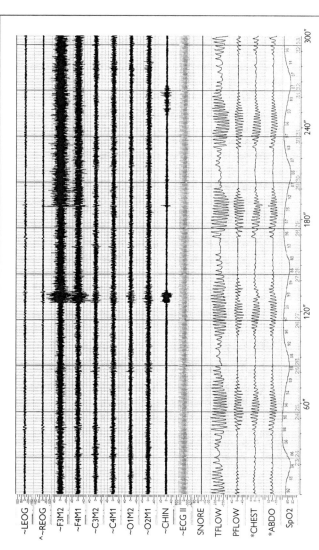

Figure 2.3 Central apneas (Cheyne-Stokes pattern). Note the crescendo-decrescendo variation in airflow (Tflow and Pflow channels) and respiratory effort (Chest and Abdo channels. Drops in oxyhemoglobin saturation (SpO2) occur with apneas. LEOG, Left electrooculogram; REOG, Right electrooculogram; F3M2, F4M1, Frontal EEG channels; C3M2, C4M1, Central EEG channels; Chin, Chin electromyogram; ECG, Electrocardiogram; Snore, Snoring; Tflow, Oral-nasal thermistor measuring airflow; Pflow, Nasal pressure transducer; Chest, Respiratory effort measured at the level of the chest using respiratory inductance plethysmography; Abdo, Respiratory effort measured at the level of the abdomen using respiratory inductance plethysmography; SpO2, Percent oxygen saturation measured with pulse oximetry.

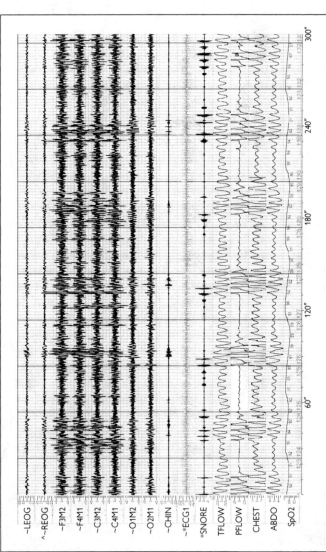

Figure 2.4 Hypopneas. Note the decrease of flow in the Tflow and Pflow channels, but the continuation of respiratory effort in the Chest and Abdo channels. Increased breathing at the termination of each hypopnea is accompanied by arousal, as indicated by increased amplitude in the EEG channels. Drops in oxyhemoglobin saturation (SpO2) occur with apneas. LEOG, Left electrooculogram; REOG, Right electrooculogram; F3M2, F4M1, Frontal EEG channels; C3M2, C4M1, Central EEG channels; Chin, Chin electromyogram; ECG, Electrocardiogram; Snore, Snoring; Tflow, Oral-nasal thermistor measuring airflow; Pflow, Nasal pressure transducer; Chest, Respiratory effort measured at the level of the chest using respiratory inductance plethysmography; Abdo, Respiratory effort measured at the level of the abdomen using respiratory inductance plethysmography; SpO2, Percent oxygen saturation measured with pulse oximetry.

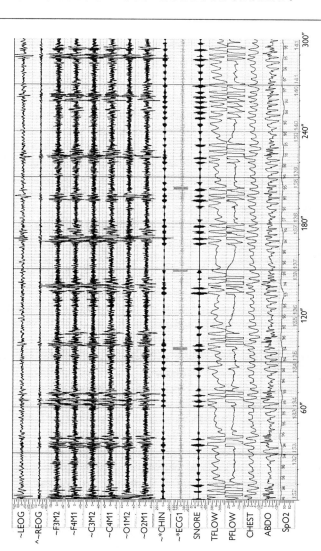

Figure 2.5 Respiratory effort-related arousals. Note that although decreased airflow (Tflow and Pflow channels) occurs and leads to arousals (increased EEG amplitude upon resumption of normal breathing), oxyhemoglobin saturation remains fairly constant. LEOG, Left electrooculogram; REOG, Right electrooculogram; F3M2, F4M1, Frontal EEG channels; C3M2, C4M1, Central EEG channels; Chin, Chin electromyogram; ECG, Electrocardiogram; Snore, Snoring; Tflow, Oral-nasal thermistor measuring airflow; Pflow, Nasal pressure transducer; Chest, Respiratory effort measured at the level of the chest using respiratory inductance plethysmography; Abdo, Respiratory effort measured at the level of the abdomen using respiratory inductance plethysmography; SpO2, Percent oxygen saturation measured with pulse oximetry.

   c.   Narrow complex tachycardia (report highest heart rate)

   d.   Wide complex tachycardia (report highest heart rate)

   e.   Atrial fibrillation

   f.   Arrhythmia

Movement Events

See Table 2.2 for PLMS scoring and Figure 2.6 for example.

1. Number of periodic limb movements during sleep (PLMS)
2. Number of PLMS with associated arousals
3. PLMS index; average number of PLMS per hour of total sleep time
4. PLMS arousal index; average number of PLMS with associated arousals per hour of total sleep time (<5)

Summary Statements

1. Sleep diagnoses based on findings
2. EEG abnormalities if present
3. ECG abnormalities if present
4. Any relevant behavioral observations
5. Comments on sleep hypnogram or architecture

The summary statement may also include recommendations for treatment or further evaluation.

Unattended Portable Monitoring

Description (Parameters Measured)

Unattended portable monitoring or home sleep studies are increasingly being used to diagnose OSA. They are less expensive, they are more acceptable to some patients, and they may be more likely to capture a "typical" night of sleep. However, they can result in technical failure if the patient is not able to apply the sensors correctly or if they become dislodged during the night.

Portable studies typically monitor significantly fewer parameters than laboratory studies and currently are used only to assess the presence of breathing disorders during sleep. At a minimum, they must record airflow, respiratory

Table 2.2 Movement Events
Periodic Limb Movement in Sleep (PLMS)
• Increase in EMG voltage of at least 8 μV above resting EMG that lasts 0.5–10 seconds • To be counted as a PLM, a limb movement must occur as part of a series of at least four consecutive limb movements. • Limb movements must occur within 5–90 seconds of each other to be considered part of the same series. • Leg movements on different legs separated by <5 seconds between movement onsets are considered as a single leg movement.
PLMS with Arousal
A limb movement is associated with an arousal when there is <0.5 seconds between the end of one event and the onset of the other, regardless of which is first.
Adapted with permission from the American Academy of Sleep Medicine. *The AASM Manual for the Scoring of Sleep and Associated Events: Rules, Terminology and Technical Specification.* Darien, IL: American Academy of Sleep Medicine, 2007.

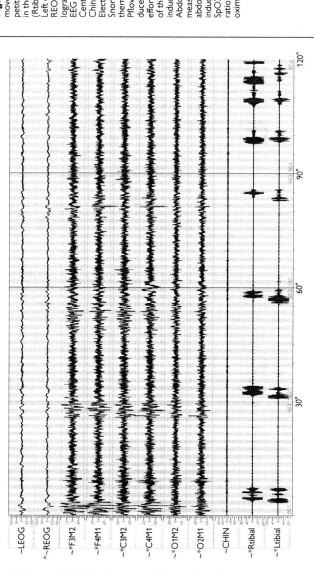

Figure 2.6 Periodic limb movements. Note the repetitive increases in activity in the leg EMG channels (Rtibial and Ltibial). LEOG, Left electrooculogram; REOG, Right electrooculogram; F3M2, F4M1, Frontal EEG channels; C3M2, C4M1, Central EEG channels; Chin, Chin electromyogram; ECG, Electrocardiogram; Snore, Snoring; Tflow, Oral-nasal thermistor measuring airflow; Pflow, Nasal pressure transducer; Chest, Respiratory effort measured at the level of the chest using respiratory inductance plethysmography; Abdo, Respiratory effort measured at the level of the abdomen using respiratory inductance plethysmography; SpO2, Percent oxygen saturation measured with pulse oximetry.

effort, and oximetry. Some studies may also add sensors to measure other variables such as position (to detect supine-dependent apnea), heart rate or heart rate variability, and snoring. Unattended portable monitoring typically does not include standard sleep staging parameters (EEG, EOG, EMG), so no sleep data are obtained. The most common type of portable study uses six channels (type 3 monitors). Portable monitoring technology continues to evolve, however, so it is likely that an increasing number of patients with sleep disorders may be able to be studied in the home setting in the future.

Indications

Portable monitoring is indicated as an alternative to in-laboratory PSG in the following cases:

1. Patients with a high probability of having moderate to severe OSA and without the following comorbidities:[13]
   a. Moderate to severe pulmonary disease, neuromuscular disease, or congestive heart failure
   b. Comorbid sleep disorders, including central sleep apnea, periodic limb movement disorder, insomnia, parasomnias, circadian rhythm sleep disorders, or narcolepsy

2. Patients with probable OSA who are unable to have in-laboratory studies because of immobility, safety, or critical illness

3. For assessment of treatment response in patients with OSA who have been treated with oral appliances, upper airway surgery, and/or weight loss

Data Included in Report

Data from portable monitoring is scored by the same criteria used for in-laboratory studies for the parameters recorded. Reports typically include the number and type of respiratory events (apneas and hypopneas) and the average number of events per hour during the recording period as an estimate of the AHI. If position monitoring is included, a supine AHI may also be included. Oximetry data (average saturation, high/low saturation, number of desaturations) is also typically provided. Heart rate data may suggest the presence of an arrhythmia.

Since sleep is not recorded, the amount of sleep time may be overestimated; it is not possible to distinguish time spent sleeping from time spent lying quietly in bed. For this reason, portable monitoring is not an ideal choice for patients with severe insomnia or for those in whom it is unclear how much time they sleep during the night.

Multiple Sleep Latency Test (MSLT)

Description

The MSLT is used to provide an objective measure of sleepiness or ability to sleep, and to detect the presence of sleep-onset REM periods for the diagnosis of narcolepsy.[14] The test is performed in the sleep laboratory, typically after a PSG, and consists of four or five nap opportunities that begin 1.5 to 3 hours after awakening in the morning and are administered every 2 hours thereafter, to assess sleep tendency across the day. To eliminate the potential effects of sleep deprivation, the patient should obtain adequate hours of sleep for a week prior to the study (documented with a sleep log or actigraphy), and a minimum of 6 hours of sleep should be obtained on the PSG on the night preceding the MSLT. Encouraging patients to sleep until they awaken spontaneously the night before the MSLT (i.e., not awakened for the convenience of the technologist in the morning) will reduce the number of false-positive MSLTs in patients with longer sleep requirements. For example, a patient who requires 10 or more hours of sleep going into an MSLT after only 6 hours of nocturnal sleep will likely appear to be excessively sleepy.

Patients taking stimulants should ideally have these tapered and discontinued for at least 2 weeks prior to the study. REM sleep-suppressing medications (such as most antidepressants) should also be tapered and discontinued, if possible, for a minimum of 2 weeks but preferably for at least 4 weeks for drugs with long half-lives, such as fluoxetine; abrupt or recent discontinuation can result in REM sleep rebound and sleep-onset REM periods.

The MSLT is administered under standardized conditions. The bedroom must be dark and quiet. Drug screening should be performed on the morning of the study if clinically indicated. Smoking should be stopped at least 30 minutes before each nap. Patients should not engage in vigorous physical activity, use caffeine, or be exposed to bright light during the testing day. Patients are given standardized instructions to lie quietly and try to sleep before every nap. The nap opportunity is terminated after 20 minutes if no sleep occurs, or 15 minutes after the first epoch of any stage of sleep.

Fewer parameters are typically recorded on an MSLT than on a PSG; the parameters recorded include EEG, EOG, EMG, and ECG.

Indications
The MSLT is indicated or may be considered in the following situations:[14]
1. Suspected narcolepsy
2. Idiopathic hypersomnia

Repeat testing is indicated when:
1. Initial testing may have been affected by extraneous circumstances or inappropriate conditions
2. Initial testing yielded ambiguous or uninterpretable findings
3. Initial testing was negative in a patient with strong suspicion of having narcolepsy

Data Included in Report
The test is scored as the average latency to sleep onset across the four or five naps, with a score of 20 minutes given to any nap in which sleep does not occur. A sleep-onset REM period is defined as the occurrence of REM sleep at any time during the nap.

The MSLT report includes the following parameters at a minimum:
1. Start and end times for each nap
2. Latency from lights-out to the first epoch of sleep
3. Mean sleep latency of all nap opportunities
4. Number of sleep-onset REM periods
5. Although not required, including data from the previous night's sleep (e.g., total sleep time, sleep efficiency, sleep latency, and REM sleep latency) is helpful for interpretation.

Accepted normative values for the MSLT are not available, and there is significant overlap between normal populations and those with sleep disorders.[15] In general, patients with narcolepsy and other disorders of excessive sleepiness will have mean sleep latencies of less than 8 minutes (and often <5 minutes), however.

Maintenance of Wakefulness Test (MWT)

Description

Whereas the MSLT assesses the ability to fall asleep, the MWT is used to document the ability of a patient to remain awake in low-stimulus situations. The MWT consists of four test opportunities, each lasting 40 minutes and administered across the day similarly to the MSLT (e.g., starting 1.5–3 hours after awakening and every 2 hours thereafter). Sleep logs should be kept for 1 week prior to testing, and PSG may be performed the previous night, depending on the clinical situation.

The tests are performed in a darkened room (light level no more than 0.13 lux at the cornea), with the patient sitting comfortably in the bed with the head supported by a pillow. The patient is instructed to sit still, look straight ahead, and attempt to remain awake. Each trial lasts 40 minutes if no sleep occurs, or is terminated after at least three consecutive epochs of stage N1 or 1 epoch of any other stage of sleep. Parameters recorded are the same as the MSLT (EEG, EOG, EMG, ECG).

Indications

The MWT is indicated to assess an individual's ability to remain awake when this may represent a potential personal or public safety issue (e.g., individuals who are being treated for sleep apnea or narcolepsy but work at jobs in which falling asleep could be hazardous). The MWT may also be helpful to assess treatment response in patients with disorders of excessive sleepiness.

Data Included in Report

The MWT is scored as the mean sleep latency across the four trials, with a score of 40 minutes for trials in which no sleep occurs. Other parameters included in the report are the following:
1. Start and stop times for each trial
2. Sleep latency for each trial
3. Total sleep time in each trial
4. Stages of sleep achieved in each trial
5. Mean sleep latency for the four trials

There are not accepted norms for interpreting the MWT, and there is significant overlap between normals and patients with sleep disorders.[15] MWT scores also increase with age; values of less than 8 minutes probably represent pathological sleepiness, as on the MSLT. However, an individual's sleep latency on the MSLT will generally be shorter than on the MWT. Mean values for normal individuals are at least 30 minutes; for individuals in whom safety is a consideration, a value of 40 minutes is desirable.

Actigraphy

Description (Parameters Measured)

Actigraphy involves wearing a wristwatch-like device (actigraph) to record movement over periods of days to weeks (Fig. 2.7A and 2.7B).[16] Movement data

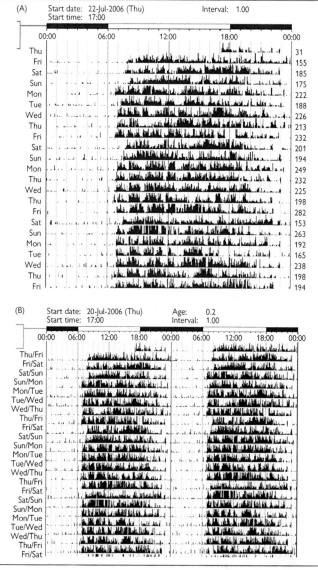

Figure 2.7 (A) A typical actigraphy display. Each horizontal line represents one 24-hour period, and vertical lines represent the sum of activity for each 1 minute of that day. This example shows someone with a very regular lifestyle. Activity is markedly reduced from about 11 p.m. each day (bedtime) until about 7 a.m. (weekdays) and 7 to 8 a.m. (weekends) when the subject gets up; in between these two times we assume the subject is asleep. There is lower activity in the evening when the subject's activities were watching TV or gardening. (B) A double plot of the same actigraphy display. Thus, each 24-hour period is plotted twice, first on the right and then on the line below on the left. This sort of plot is useful to show shifts of sleep–wake pattern in disruptions of circadian rhythm.

are summed over periods of time of up to 1 minute for a minimum of 3 days but preferably at least 1 week, particularly for circadian rhythm disorders. Patients keep a sleep log simultaneously to record parameters such as when they go to bed at night (to allow for calculation of sleep latency) and daytime activities such as napping or exercise. Some actigraphs also record light exposure, which may provide useful clinical information for some disorders, including circadian rhythm disorders and insomnia.

Indications

Actigraphy may be used to document patterns of rest and activity in the following situations:

1. Normal, healthy individuals
2. Individuals suspected of having circadian rhythm sleep disorders
3. When PSG is not available, it may be used to estimate total sleep time in patients with OSA in conjunction with monitoring of respiratory events
4. Patients with insomnia
5. Patients with hypersomnia
6. To assess response to treatment in patients with circadian rhythm sleep disorders and insomnia
7. To document sleep patterns in special populations, including older adults living in the community or in nursing homes, or in infants or children

Data Included in Report

Actigraphy reports typically include total sleep time each day, time of sleep onset and waking time, and nap times. If sleep log data are available, sleep latency and sleep efficiency may be calculated as well.

References

1. American Academy of Sleep Medicine. *International Classification of Sleep Disorders: Diagnostic and Coding Manual,* 2nd ed. Westchester, IL: American Academy of Sleep Medicine, 2005.

2. Chesson A, Jr., Hartse K, Anderson WM, et al. Practice parameters for the evaluation of chronic insomnia. An American Academy of Sleep Medicine report. Standards of Practice Committee of the American Academy of Sleep Medicine. *Sleep.* 2000 Mar 15;23(2):237–41.

3. Johns MW. A new method for measuring daytime sleepiness: the Epworth sleepiness scale. *Sleep.* 1991 Dec;14(6):540–5.

4. Bastien CH, Vallieres A, Morin CM. Validation of the Insomnia Severity Index as an outcome measure for insomnia research. *Sleep Med.* 2001 Jul;2(4):297–307.

5. Krupp LB, LaRocca NG, Muir-Nash J, et al. The Fatigue Severity Scale. Application to patients with multiple sclerosis and systemic lupus erythematosus. *Arch Neurol.* 1989 Oct;46(10):1121–3.

6. International Restless Legs Syndrome Study Group. Validation of the International Restless Legs Syndrome Study Group rating scale for restless legs syndrome. *Sleep Med.* 2003 Mar;4(2):121–32.

7. Netzer NC, Stoohs RA, Netzer CM, et al. Using the Berlin Questionnaire to identify patients at risk for the sleep apnea syndrome. *Ann Intern Med.* 1999 Oct 5;131(7):485–91.

8. Horne JA, Ostberg O. A self-assessment questionnaire to determine morningness-eveningness in human circadian rhythms. *Int J Chronobiol*. 1976;4(2):97—110.

9. Beck AT, Steer RA, Brown GK. *Manual for the Beck Depression Inventory*. San Antonio, TX: Psychological Corporation, 1996.

10. Radloff LS. The CES-D Scale: A self-report depression scale for research in the general population. *Applied Psychological Measurement*. 1977;1:385–401.

11. American Academy of Sleep Medicine. *The AASM Manual for the Scoring of Sleep and Associated Events: Rules, Terminology and Technical Specification*. Westchester, IL: American Academy of Sleep Medicine, 2007.

12. Kushida CA, Littner MR, Morgenthaler T, et al. Practice parameters for the indications for polysomnography and related procedures: an update for 2005. *Sleep*. 2005 Apr 1;28(4):499–521.

13. Collop NA, Anderson WM, Boehlecke B, et al. Clinical guidelines for the use of unattended portable monitors in the diagnosis of obstructive sleep apnea in adult patients. Portable Monitoring Task Force of the American Academy of Sleep Medicine. *J Clin Sleep Med*. 2007 Dec 15;3(7):737–47.

14. Littner MR, Kushida C, Wise M, et al. Practice parameters for clinical use of the multiple sleep latency test and the maintenance of wakefulness test. *Sleep*. 2005 Jan 1;28(1):113–21.

15. Arand D, Bonnet M, Hurwitz T, et al. The clinical use of the MSLT and MWT. *Sleep*. 2005 Jan 1;28(1):123–44.

16. Littner M, Kushida CA, Anderson WM, et al. Practice parameters for the role of actigraphy in the study of sleep and circadian rhythms: an update for 2002. *Sleep*. 2003 May 1;26(3):337–41.

Chapter 3

Insomnia

Description

Insomnia is one of the most common problems encountered in medical practice. As a symptom, insomnia refers to sleep difficulties consisting of insufficient
quantity or quality of sleep that may accompany other medical or psychiatric disorders, or occur as responses to psychosocial stressors. Insomnia as a
disorder includes not only complaints of sleep disturbance, but also daytime
dysfunction. Specific symptoms include difficulty falling asleep at the beginning
of the night, frequent and/or prolonged awakenings during the sleep period,
waking up earlier in the morning than desired, and the perception that the sleep
obtained is not restorative or refreshing. Diagnosis of an insomnia disorder also
requires that there are significant daytime symptoms associated with the sleep
disturbance; these include fatigue or sleepiness, problems with attention and
concentration, mood disturbance, impaired function at school or work, physical
symptoms, and worries about sleep. Importantly, insomnia differs from sleep
deprivation in that the lack of sleep is not due to inadequate opportunity to
sleep; not infrequently, insomnia patients report spending increased time in bed
in their attempts to get enough sleep. Criteria for the diagnosis of an insomnia
disorder are listed in Table 3.1.

Insomnia can be defined as acute or chronic, depending on its duration.
Acute insomnia usually lasts only days or up to a few weeks and typically occurs
in response to various stressors, such as environmental factors (e.g., sleeping
in a strange environment, noise), illness, pain, or other psychosocial stressors.
Once the precipitating factor is eliminated or resolved, sleep frequently returns
to normal. However, in some cases, sleep disturbance may persist and lead to
chronic insomnia.

Insomnia that lasts at least 1 month is defined as chronic. The majority of
individuals with chronic insomnia, however, report that their sleep problem has
lasted for years.[1] As a result, distinguishing between acute and chronic insomnia
in the clinical setting is usually not difficult.

Chronic insomnia often begins in early adulthood and may be initially triggered by a stressful event. Some individuals, however, may report an almost
life-long history of poor sleep without a clear precipitant or onset. Chronic
insomnia frequently has a waxing and waning course, with exacerbations connected to recurrent stressful events. Night-to-night variability is also common,
and the relative severity of specific symptoms may change over time.

Table 3.1 Criteria for Insomnia Diagnosis (ICSD-2)

A. One or more of the following symptoms:
- Difficulty initiating sleep
- Difficulty maintaining sleep
- Waking up too early
- Nonrestorative sleep

B. Sleep difficulty occurs despite adequate opportunity for sleep

C. At least one of the following daytime symptoms related to the nighttime sleep difficulty reported:
- Fatigue/malaise
- Attention, concentration, or memory impairment
- Social/vocational dysfunction or poor school performance
- Mood disturbance/irritability
- Daytime sleepiness
- Motivation/energy/initiative reduction
- Proneness for errors/accidents
- Tension headaches and/or gastrointestinal symptoms
- Concerns or worries about sleep

Adapted with permission from the American Academy of Sleep Medicine. *International Classification of Sleep Disorders: Diagnostic and Coding Manual*, 2nd ed. Darien, IL: American Academy of Sleep Medicine, 2005.

Chronic insomnia is further subdivided into primary or comorbid types. At least 80% of cases of chronic insomnia occur in patients with medical or psychiatric disorders.[2] Previously, this had been called secondary insomnia, since it was presumed that insomnia was caused by the other disorder(s). It is now recognized that the relationships between insomnia and other disorders are more complex; insomnia is not only exacerbated by a large number of medical and psychiatric conditions, but it can also aggravate and/or lead to poorer outcomes in these conditions.[3,4] Furthermore, comorbid insomnia does not necessarily remit with or respond to the same treatments as the associated medical or psychiatric condition. Only about 10% to 20% of cases are considered primary insomnia, meaning that they do not appear to be related to any other medical or psychiatric conditions, medication effects, or substance use. Patients with primary insomnia often report longstanding problems with sleep, sometimes dating back into childhood.

Despite its high prevalence, insomnia is often undiagnosed and/or untreated. In part, this may be due to a lack of awareness by patients or healthcare providers of the health consequences of insomnia. Chronic insomnia has been linked with impairments ranging from poorer concentration, memory problems, increased absenteeism, decreased job performance, increased accidents and falls, and increased healthcare costs. More recent data suggest that insomnia may increase the risk for the development of hypertension and depression.[5–7]

Epidemiology

Estimates of the prevalence of insomnia vary based on the definitions used. For example, symptoms of insomnia are commonly experienced and probably affect over half of the U.S. population over the course of a year. Insomnia with daytime consequences has been estimated to affect about 10% to 15% of the general population, according to a number of epidemiological studies performed in the United States, Europe, and Asia.[6,8,9] Relatively few studies have assessed the epidemiology of strictly defined insomnia disorder in the general population, but the estimate obtained from these studies is about 6%.[10]

Certain populations are at greater risk for insomnia.[2] Women are almost 1.5 times more likely than men to have insomnia, which has been attributed to the greater risk they have for depression. Their risk increases further at the onset of menopause. Elderly people report sleep complaints more frequently than younger individuals, at least in part because they tend to suffer from more illnesses, including other sleep disorders. Adults who have lost their partners through death or divorce are also at increased risk. Insomnia appears to have a familial component as well, although specific genes for insomnia have not been identified. Risk factors and common comorbidities for insomnia are shown in Table 3.2.

Table 3.2 Insomnia Risk Factors and Comorbidities

Age (greater prevalence in older individuals)

Female gender (especially post- and perimenopausal)

Divorce/separation/widowhood

Family history

Psychiatric illness

    Adjustment disorders

    Anxiety disorders (e.g., generalized anxiety, panic disorder, post-traumatic stress disorder)

    Eating disorders (e.g., anorexia nervosa, bulimia nervosa)

    Mood disorders (e.g., major depressive disorder, bipolar disorder)

    Schizophrenia

    Substance abuse disorders

Medical conditions, particularly multiple conditions

    Cancer

    Cardiovascular disease

    Chronic pain syndromes

    Dementia

    Dermatological disorders

    Endocrine disorders

    Fibromyalgia

    Gastroesophageal reflux disease

    Infectious disease

    Inflammatory bowel disease

(continued)

Table 3.2 (continued)

Parkinson's disease
Perimenopause
Pulmonary disorders
Rheumatological disorders
Seizure disorders
Urological disorders

Primary sleep disorders
    Circadian rhythm disorders
    Parasomnias
    Periodic movement disorder
    Restless legs syndrome
    Sleep apnea

Substance use/abuse
    Alcohol
    Caffeine
    Stimulants
    Tobacco

Medications
    Antidepressants (SSRIs, bupropion)
    Antihypertensives
    Bronchodilators
    Corticosteroids
    Decongestants (phenylpropanolamine, pseudoephedrine)
    Diuretics
    Quinidine
    Stimulants
    Theophylline

Clinical populations have much higher rates of insomnia than the general population. In general, the more medical problems a patient has, the more likely he or she is to have insomnia. Insomnia rates are probably greatest in psychiatric populations because acute psychiatric disorders correlate highly with insomnia. Even in primary care settings, the most common comorbid conditions with insomnia are depression and anxiety disorders.

Insomnia is not only comorbid with most psychiatric disorders, but it also is predictive of new onset or recurrence of psychiatric illness, particularly mood disorders.[11] Furthermore, in patients with depression, sleep disturbance is one of the last symptoms to remit and often persists despite treatment of the underlying mood disorder. Insomnia also appears to contribute to chronic pain conditions, in that the daytime experience of pain severity has been associated with the degree of insomnia on the preceding night in some studies.

There is now emerging evidence that treatment of insomnia may help to improve some of its comorbid conditions. For example, some studies have suggested that depression may remit more quickly when patients are treated for insomnia along with specific treatment for their depression.[12,13]

Pathophysiology

Insomnia patients tend to show evidence of physiological hyperarousal,[14–16] as indicated by increased body temperature, heart rate, and metabolic rate before and during the sleep period. They also tend to show increased fast (beta) activity during the sleep EEG and decreased slow-wave sleep or slow-wave activity during sleep. There is also evidence of increased activity of the hypothalamic–pituitary–adrenal axis, with increased levels of catecholamines, cortisol, and ACTH. Neuroimaging studies have demonstrated increased brain metabolic rates during waking and sleep, and increased activation in arousal systems during sleep in insomnia patients in comparison to normal controls.

Psychological and behavioral factors also contribute to insomnia. Insomnia patients tend to be generally more reactive to stresses and have more worries and intrusive thoughts prior to sleep. Over time, they may become conditioned to have negative associations to the sleep environment and bedtime, leading to further anxiety and hyperarousal. They frequently develop maladaptive responses to their insomnia in an effort to get more sleep, such as napping during the day, which further decreases the homeostatic drive to sleep at night, or increasing time in bed, which contributes to sleep fragmentation. Unfortunately, these behaviors serve to perpetuate the insomnia.

Although the specific causes of insomnia are not known, current evidence supports the theory proposed by Spielman regarding the course of insomnia.[17] Individuals are likely predisposed to develop insomnia due to genetic/biological factors that make them hyperaroused and more reactive to stress. Precipitating factors such as stressful events or illnesses may trigger the initial bout and exacerbations of insomnia. Perpetuating factors such as poor sleep habits, increased worry about sleep, and conditioned associations to the sleep environment that increase arousal contribute to maintaining insomnia. As a result, optimal treatment of chronic insomnia needs to address these various components.

Evaluation

Insomnia is a clinical diagnosis, based on patient report. It is important to assess not only the presence of specific symptoms of insomnia (see Table 3.1) but also their frequency, severity, and duration to guide evaluation and treatment. Lichstein has suggested that as a guideline for clinical trials, chronic insomnia should be defined as spending more than 30 minutes to fall asleep or more than 30 minutes awake after sleep onset at least three times per week for at least 6 months.[18] American Academy of Sleep Medicine (AASM) guidelines for the diagnosis of insomnia recommend cutoffs of total sleep time less than

6.5 hours and/or sleep efficiency of less than 85%. These criteria are also reasonable for assessing patients clinically, although the patient's perception of the severity of the sleep problem is ultimately most important in guiding further evaluation and treatment. Sleep diaries or logs can be useful in helping to define the pattern and severity of the sleep disturbance and should be filled out for a minimum of 1 week (an example is provided in Appendix 6).

Evaluation requires thorough assessment, not only of the sleep complaint, but also of any relevant comorbidities, since treatment must focus on both the insomnia and its contributing comorbid conditions. For example, patients who experience the most severe sleep difficulties may have comorbid psychiatric illnesses, particularly mood, anxiety, and psychotic disorders; they may complain primarily about their sleep, preferring to think that treating their insomnia would eliminate all their other symptoms and problems. The daytime effects and symptoms of insomnia should also be established, since resolution of daytime dysfunction is an important target outcome for assessing treatment response.

Evaluation should include documentation of the patient's sleep patterns, including bedtime routine, regularity of sleep schedule, pattern of sleep across the night, and any daytime napping. A patient's sleep history should indicate the onset and potential relationship to any concomitant illnesses or stressors; the course of the disorder, including factors that tend to exacerbate the sleep problem as well as those that make it better (e.g., vacations); and any treatments that have been attempted and the response to them.

Several self-report screening tools are available to identify and quantify insomnia. The Pittsburgh Sleep Quality Index (PSQI) is a 19-item questionnaire that takes about 5 to 10 minutes to complete and a few minutes to score (Appendix 8).[19] A global score of more than 5 (out of a total of 21 possible points) indicates significant sleep disturbance, with higher scores associated with more severe problems. The Insomnia Severity Index (ISI) consists of 7 items rated on a 0-to-4 scale and takes only minutes to complete and score (Appendix 7).[20] Scores of 8 to 14 indicate mild insomnia, 15 to 21 moderate insomnia, and 22 to 28 severe insomnia. Both of these scales have been shown to have good reliability and validity in identifying insomnia patients in general and clinical populations. They are useful not only in diagnosis but also in assessing treatment outcome. Other scales can be useful in quantifying associated symptoms such as sleepiness (Epworth Sleepiness Scale[21] [Appendix 5]) and fatigue (Fatigue Severity Index[22]); although fatigue is common in insomnia, elevated sleepiness may indicate the presence of another sleep problem, such as apnea.

Given the high comorbidity between insomnia and psychiatric disorders, all insomnia patients must be screened at a minimum for depression and anxiety. Useful screening measures include the Beck Depression Inventory or the Center for Epidemiologic Studies Depression Scale (CES-D) (Appendix 11) and the State-Trait Anxiety Inventory. History of any past psychiatric illnesses should be obtained, since significant insomnia is a risk factor for recurrence. Other medical problems can contribute to insomnia; therefore, they should be assessed and their treatment optimized. Medications used to treat psychiatric or medical problems should be evaluated regarding their potential contribution to the insomnia complaint.

The patient's use of substances that contribute to insomnia should be determined, and toxicology screening or serum drug levels should be considered if abuse is suspected. Stimulants, caffeine, and nicotine can interfere with sleep. Alcohol is frequently used in attempts to self-medicate for insomnia. Although initially it promotes sleep, it can contribute to insomnia in the latter part of the night, as blood alcohol levels drop. Chronic alcohol abuse can lead to insomnia that may persist despite prolonged abstinence from drinking.

Environmental factors such as noise, a bedroom that is too warm or cold, or an uncomfortable bed may also contribute to sleep problems. Behavioral factors such as timing and amount of exercise (too little or at the wrong times), bright light exposure near the sleep period or insufficient light during the day, shift work, or frequent travel may also play a role in perpetuating sleep problems.

Physical examination and laboratory testing should be performed based on the overall medical assessment and comorbid conditions. Although no specific testing is indicated for insomnia, common disorders that may contribute to fatigue or sleep disturbance such as hypothyroidism or anemia should be considered.

Polysomnography is not indicated for the routine assessment of insomnia and should be used only if other sleep disorders such as sleep apnea or sleep-related movement disorders are suspected. It may also be considered in patients who are resistant to treatment or who have histories of violent behavior or self-injury during sleep. Actigraphy is also not indicated for the initial assessment of insomnia, but it may be useful if sleep diary data are not considered to be reliable. Recommended diagnostic evaluation of insomnia is provided in Table 3.3.

Table 3.3 Evaluation of Insomnia[23]
Sleep complaint
Symptoms
Difficulty falling asleep
Number and duration of nocturnal awakenings
Early morning awakening
Nonrestorative sleep
Onset
Duration
Frequency
Severity
Course
Precipitants and perpetuating factors (e.g., stress, pain, illness)
Other sleep-related symptoms
Respiratory (e.g., snoring, witnessed apneas, waking gasping for breath)
Motor (e.g., restless legs, kicking/twitching during sleep, sleepwalking)
Other medical (e.g., pain, reflux, urinary frequency)
Psychological (e.g., worries about sleep, thoughts/emotions during periods of waking)

(continued)

Table 3.3 (continued)

Behaviors related to sleep

    Bedtime and time required to fall asleep, wake-up time

    Regularity of schedule (weekdays/weekends)

    Pre-sleep activities

    Behaviors during nocturnal arousals

    Bedroom environment

    Napping

    Exercise

Daytime function

    Sleepiness versus fatigue

    Daytime consequences (see Table 3.1)

Medication and substance use

    Over-the-counter agents

    Prescription medications

    Recreational drugs, including alcohol and tobacco

    Caffeine use

Prior treatment history and response

Medical history and examination

Psychiatric history and examination

Sleep disorder screening

Sleep log or diary (at least 1 week)

Actigraphy if sleep log data are unreliable

Polysomnography only in cases of suspected sleep apnea, movement disorder, or parasomnia

Consider use of rating scales to assess baseline severity and assess outcome

    Insomnia Severity Index or Pittsburgh Sleep Quality Index (insomnia severity)

    Epworth Sleepiness Scale (sleepiness)

    Fatigue Severity Scale (fatigue)

    Beck Depression Inventory (depression)

    State-Trait Anxiety Inventory (anxiety)

    Short Form Health Survey (SF-36) (quality of life)

    Dysfunctional Beliefs and Attitudes about Sleep (DBAS) Questionnaire (negative cognitions about sleep)

Source: Schutte-Rodin S, Broch L, Buysse D, et al. Clinical guideline for the evaluation and management of chronic insomnia in adults. *J Clin Sleep Med.* 2008 Oct 15;4(5):487–504.

Diagnosis

Insomnia may be acute or chronic. Acute insomnia is usually associated with an identifiable stressor and lasts no more than 3 months, and usually less; it resolves when the stressor is removed. Chronic insomnia lasts a minimum of 1 month, but most individuals with chronic insomnia in the general population report symptoms lasting for a year or more.[1] Insomnia can also exist as a primary disorder or comorbid with other conditions. Primary insomnias can include acute or short-term insomnia related to a stressor (adjustment insomnia) or more chronic conditions such as psychophysiological insomnia (learned or conditioned insomnia), paradoxical insomnia (subjective insomnia or sleep state misperception), idiopathic insomnia (childhood onset or life-long insomnia), insomnia related to inadequate sleep hygiene, and behavioral insomnia of childhood. Comorbid insomnias include those associated with other disorders that may induce or exacerbate sleep problems, such as insomnia due to a drug or substance or insomnia due to a medical condition or mental disorder. Children may develop behavioral insomnia, characterized by difficulties getting to sleep or returning to sleep; this is characterized either by refusal to go to bed and/or behaviors that prolong going to bed and may be related to inabilities of caregivers to appropriately set limits in some cases. Specific insomnia diagnoses and their associated features are listed in Table 3.4.[24]

Table 3.4 Insomnia Disorders
Adjustment insomnia (acute insomnia)
Associated with an identifiable stressor
Resolves with removal of or adaptation to the stressor
Duration <3 months
Psychophysiological insomnia
Conditioned insomnia associated with heightened arousal in bed
Symptoms may include anxiety about sleep; difficulty falling asleep in bed at bedtime, while easily falling asleep in low-stimulus settings when not planning to sleep; ability to fall asleep better away from home; increased mental arousal in bed; increased physical arousal/tension in bed
Duration at least 1 month
Paradoxical insomnia
Patient reports chronically getting little to no sleep at night and no daytime napping.
Patient reports awareness of surroundings and/or conscious thought/rumination throughout most of the night.
Actigraphy or polysomnography data show significantly greater amounts of sleep than reported by the patient.
No symptoms of sleep deprivation reported
Duration at least 1 month
Idiopathic insomnia
Persistent, life-long insomnia beginning in childhood
No identifiable cause
Insomnia due to mental disorder
Patient has a diagnosed mental disorder, with insomnia more severe than typically occurs in association with the disorder.
Insomnia symptoms are temporally related to the mental disorder, although they may appear prior to onset and persist after remission of the disorder.
Duration at least 1 month

(continued)

Table 3.4 (continued)

Inadequate sleep hygiene

Insomnia due to poor sleep hygiene practices, such as irregular sleep schedules, use of substances (alcohol, caffeine, nicotine) before bed, engaging in activating or stimulating activities before bedtime, use of the bed for activities other than sleep, and/or uncomfortable sleep environment

Duration at least 1 month

Behavioral insomnia of childhood

Childhood insomnia with problems related to sleep associations (problematic sleep-onset associations, with falling asleep an extended process requiring special conditions, and sleep onset delayed if the associated conditions are not present), or limit-setting issues (child has difficulty getting to sleep, stalls or refuses to go to sleep, and/or the caregiver is unable to set appropriate limits for the child)

Insomnia due to drug or substance use

Insomnia caused by either (1) abuse of or dependence on a drug or substance that can disturb sleep through use or withdrawal or (2) ingestion, use, or exposure to food, medication, or toxin that can disrupt sleep

Duration at least 1 month

Insomnia due to a medical condition

Patient has a diagnosed medical condition that can disrupt sleep (e.g., chronic pain syndrome, benign prostatic hypertrophy).

Insomnia symptoms are temporally related to the course of the medical condition.

Duration at least 1 month

Insomnia not due to substance or known physiologic condition, unspecified (nonorganic insomnia, NOS)

Insomnia thought to be related to underlying mental disorder or behavioral factors but does not meet criteria for another insomnia diagnosis

Physiologic (organic) insomnia, unspecified

Insomnia thought to be related to underlying medical disorder or substance use/exposure but does not meet criteria for another insomnia diagnosis

Adapted with permission from the American Academy of Sleep Medicine. *International Classification of Sleep Disorders: Diagnostic and Coding Manual*, 2nd ed. Darien, IL: American Academy of Sleep Medicine, 2005.

Insomnia complaints can also be prominent in several other sleep disorders. Up to half of sleep apnea patients may complain of significant sleep disturbance; these sleep complaints are more common among women and those with anxiety or mood problems.[25] Restless legs syndrome can contribute to difficulties falling asleep or remaining asleep, whereas periodic limb movement disorder can cause sleep fragmentation and arousals during sleep, thus decreasing sleep quality. Patients with circadian rhythm disorders can have profound insomnia when the desired sleep schedule does not match their internal circadian rhythm, such as night-shift workers who try to sleep during the day, or in individuals with delayed sleep phase syndrome who are unable to fall asleep until well past the desired bedtime but then are unable to wake up in time for work or school in the morning. In particular, patients who have insomnia with profound daytime sleepiness should be assessed for other sleep disorders, since insomnia patients typically have trouble sleeping at any time of day, although they can complain of severe fatigue. On the other hand, individuals who complain about their inability to get what they feel is a sufficient amount of sleep at night compared to their peers but do not have any daytime complaints as a result may simply be short sleepers (i.e., they require less than the average 8 hours of sleep per night) and do not require treatment.

Treatment

Treatment of insomnia should proceed in a stepwise fashion, as indicated in Table 3.5. The first step in treatment is to eliminate or at least minimize comorbid medical illnesses, psychiatric conditions, and/or other primary sleep disorders identified in the evaluation that may be contributing to insomnia. For example, symptoms such as pain, nocturia, or vasomotor symptoms (hot flashes) that interfere with sleep should be reduced as much as possible. Symptomatic psychiatric disorders should be treated, including referral to mental health providers if needed. Disorders such as sleep apnea or restless legs should generally be treated first, as insomnia caused by these may remit without additional therapy. Medications, including over-the-counter agents, should be reviewed and those that may be interfering with sleep should be eliminated if possible, or their use avoided near bedtime.

Cognitive and Behavioral Therapies

All patients with insomnia should be instructed in proper sleep hygiene (Table 3.6). Although sleep hygiene alone is not considered sufficient treatment for insomnia, it is an important first step to ensure that patients are not engaging in behaviors that are likely to worsen their sleep difficulties. Sleep hygiene rules are generally intended to reinforce the circadian and homeostatic drives to sleep (e.g., by having consistent bedtimes and wake-up times and avoiding napping), decreasing arousal in bed (e.g., having a relaxing bedtime routine and eliminating activities other than sleep or sex in bed), and avoiding substances or activities that interfere with sleep (e.g., caffeine, alcohol, exercise, or bright light exposure near bedtime).

Table 3.5 Treatment of Insomnia
1. Treat any underlying cause(s)/comorbid conditions (psychiatric disorders, pain, apnea, other medical or sleep disorders, medications, substance use/abuse)
2. Promote good sleep habits (sleep hygiene instruction)
3. Consider cognitive behavior therapy (available data suggest similar efficacy in comorbid and primary insomnia)
4. Consider medications to improve sleep

Table 3.6 Sleep Hygiene Instructions

Reinforce homeostatic and circadian drives for sleep:

1. Maintain a regular bedtime and wake-up time.
2. Avoid napping.
3. Exercise regularly, but not within several hours of bedtime or early in the morning if early awakening is a problem.
4. Increase bright light exposure during the day and minimize at night.

Optimize sleep environment:

1. Bedroom should be dark, quiet, comfortable, and slightly cool in temperature.
2. Use bed only for sleep and sex.
3. Eliminate televisions, computers, etc. from bedroom.
4. Minimize noise in bedroom; consider a white noise machine to mask background noise if necessary.

Eliminate factors that interfere with sleep:

1. Have a relaxing routine prior to bedtime for at least 1 hour to decrease arousal; avoid stimulating or stressful activities prior to bedtime.
2. Do not watch the clock at night.
3. Eliminate caffeine and nicotine if possible; at a minimum, do not use for at least 6–8 hours prior to bedtime.
4. Drink alcohol in moderation and try to avoid use for at least several hours prior to bedtime.
5. Do not consume excessive fluids for at least 6 hours before bedtime.
6. Do not go to bed hungry or immediately after a large meal.

A number of behavioral treatments are helpful in the treatment of chronic insomnia, including both primary and comorbid types.[26] **Stimulus control** is designed to help the patient associate the bedroom and bedtime with sleep rather than distress and frustration in anticipation of another night of insomnia.[27] The patient must adhere to specific instructions that are intended to minimize the amount of time spent lying awake in bed—for instance, leaving the bed after 20 minutes when unable to sleep (Table 3.7). Patients may be concerned about not getting sufficient sleep for the first nights with this therapy, but as their sleep debt builds up, they should fall asleep closer to the desired bedtime. This is sometimes a difficult therapy for patients to follow, since failure to follow the rules strictly, such as by lying in bed ruminating, or sleeping in late, can diminish success.

Relaxation training is probably the most common behavioral approach, since it is frequently used for a variety of non-sleep disorders such as anxiety and most behavioral therapists are familiar with it. Self-help books and tapes are also readily available. There are two general categories of relaxation training: physical and mental. Physical interventions include progressive muscle relaxation and breathing exercises. Mental relaxation approaches include various forms of meditation and guided imagery. Relaxation is primarily intended to reduce arousal in bed.

Table 3.7 Cognitive and Behavioral Treatments for Insomnia

Stimulus Control Instructions

1. Go to bed only when sleepy.
2. If unable to fall asleep within about 20 minutes, or if experiencing increased arousal in bed, get out of bed and engage in a relaxing activity (e.g., reading) until feeling sleepy.
3. Repeat Steps 1 and 2 until sleep occurs.
4. Wake up at the same time each morning, even if total sleep time was less than desired.
5. Do not nap during the day.

Relaxation Training Approaches

For somatic arousal:

1. Progressive muscle relaxation
2. Abdominal breathing
3. Biofeedback
4. Autogenic training (creates warm, heavy, relaxed feeling throughout body)

For cognitive arousal:

1. Guided imagery
2. Meditation
3. Thought stopping

Sleep Restriction Instructions

1. Have patient keep a sleep log for 1–2 weeks and determine mean total sleep time per day.
2. Set bedtime and waking time to obtain sleep amount determined in Step 1 with an 85% sleep efficiency (sleep efficiency = total sleep time/time in bed × 100%). Time in bed may not be set lower than 5 hours.
3. On a weekly basis, increase time in bed by 15–20 minutes/night if sleep efficiency is >85%, decrease time in bed by 15–20 minutes/night for sleep efficiency <80%; no change if sleep efficiency 80–85%.
4. Repeat Step 3 on a weekly basis.

Cognitive Behavior Therapy for Insomnia (CBT-I)

Components include:

1. Cognitive therapy, aimed at changing dysfunctional beliefs and attitudes about sleep (e.g., create more realistic expectations, decrease catastrophizing about effects of insomnia)
2. Behavioral therapy, which may include stimulus control, sleep restriction, relaxation therapy

Sleep restriction therapy is intended to improve sleep consolidation by minimizing time in bed so that the resulting sleep debt will increase the homeostatic drive to sleep.[28] Many insomnia patients will compensate for lost sleep by increasing time in bed: going to bed early, staying in bed later, and lying down during the day to obtain more sleep. However, spending too much time in bed can actually fragment sleep and worsen insomnia. In sleep restriction therapy, patients are instructed to keep a sleep log or diary for at least 1 week, and are then instructed to decrease the time they spend in bed to the average number of hours of reported sleep, but not less than 5 hours per night. They must continue to maintain the sleep diary throughout the treatment period so that their sleep efficiency (number of hours of sleep divided by hours in bed) can be calculated (Fig. 3.1). As their sleep consolidation improves, the amount of time they are allowed to spend in bed is gradually increased. Sleep restriction should not be used in patients with a history of seizures or bipolar disorder, as sleep deprivation may lower the seizure threshold and induce mania.

Cognitive behavior therapy is a multimodal approach that combines one or more behavioral interventions (e.g., sleep hygiene, stimulus control, sleep restriction, relaxation training) with cognitive therapy for insomnia. Patients with chronic insomnia often develop dysfunctional attitudes about sleep, such as the feeling that they "cannot function" without a certain amount of sleep, or that lack of sleep will cause serious harm to them; as a result, they become

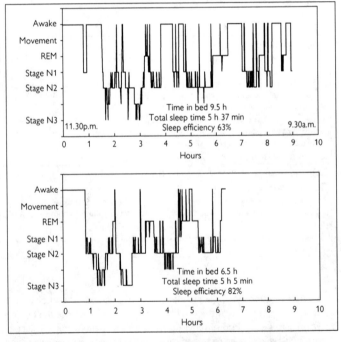

Figure 3.1 Bedtime restriction improves sleep efficiency. In the upper hynogram, the patient spent 9.5 hours in bed, slept for about 5.5 hours, and had a sleep efficiency of 63%. Restricting time in bed to 6.5 hours reduced sleep to just over 5 hours but increased sleep efficiency to 82%, and the patient reported an improvement in sleep quality.

more worried about their sleep and more aroused in the sleep environment. These beliefs are challenged and the patient is encouraged to adopt more realistic assessments.

Paradoxical intention is based on the premise that in some cases insomnia may be related to "performance anxiety" regarding falling asleep. The patient is instructed to try to stay awake while in bed at night rather than "try" to sleep, with the goal of decreasing bedtime worry. **Biofeedback** approaches include monitoring parameters such as temperature, brain wave frequencies, or EMG; they are not used frequently because of the expense of the equipment and the difficulty some patients have learning the techniques.

Behavioral treatments for insomnia are effective, particularly in treating sleep onset insomnia and improving the overall quality of sleep.[29] They can also increase total sleep and decrease the number and duration of awakenings during the sleep period. The magnitude of these effects on sleep quality and awakenings is comparable to that produced by hypnotic medication.[30] Furthermore, behavioral treatments can have long-lasting effects, with studies demonstrating persistent improvements in sleep over periods as long as 2 to 3 years in those who continue to adhere to them. However, they are greatly underused for a variety of reasons, including insufficient training of primary care providers, lack of trained behavioral health specialists or sleep specialists, and poor motivation by patients to practice behavioral techniques. Behavioral treatments are more time-consuming for both patients and healthcare providers but have the advantage of long-term efficacy and none of the side effects associated with use of medications for sleep. Healthcare providers should be able to treat many patients effectively using the approaches described above, alone or in combination with pharmacotherapy. Complex or treatment-resistant cases may require referral to a behavioral sleep specialist. Guidelines for the choice of behavioral treatments are listed in Table 3.8.

Table 3.8 Psychological and Behavioral Interventions for Insomnia[31]
Recommended (Standards)
Stimulus control
Relaxation training
Cognitive behavior therapy
Recommended (Guidelines)
Sleep restriction
Multicomponent therapy (without cognitive therapy)
Paradoxical intention
Biofeedback
Source: Peterson MJ, Benca RM. Sleep in mood disorders. *Psychiatric Clin North Am.* 2006 Dec;29(4):1009–32; abstract ix.

Pharmacologic Therapy

Medications used to treat insomnia include over-the-counter (OTC) agents, hypnotics that are approved by the U.S. Food and Drug Administration (FDA) for the treatment of insomnia, and other prescription agents used off-label for their sleep-promoting effects.[32] Individuals with insomnia, particularly those with less severe complaints, commonly use OTC agents as a first-line approach. Patients may also self-medicate with alcohol, but this should be actively discouraged since acute use can cause fragmentation of sleep later in the night, and chronic use can lead to chronic insomnia and, potentially, to alcohol abuse or addiction.

OTC Agents

Most OTC sleep agents contain antihistamines (either diphenhydramine or doxylamine) that antagonize type 1 histamine (H1) receptors in the brain. These agents can be sedating in some individuals, although there are relatively few data regarding their use in insomnia; they can have paradoxical effects and cause excitation in young children or the elderly. Furthermore, they can cause rapid tolerance and rebound insomnia and may not be effective for chronic use.[33] They can have significant side effects, including daytime drowsiness or hangover, paradoxical agitation, anticholinergic effects, cardiotoxicity, and potential exacerbation of restless legs.

Other frequently used OTC agents include melatonin, a hormone produced by the pineal gland, and valerian, prepared from the root of the plant *Valeriana officinalis*; neither is regulated by the FDA. Melatonin is rapidly absorbed and has a short half-life of about 1 hour. The mechanism of action of valerian is not specifically known, but it may act by increasing GABA transmission. Relatively few adverse events have been reported with either melatonin or valerian, but there are also limited data supporting their efficacy for insomnia. A recent meta-analysis has suggested that valerian may produce some subjective improvement in insomnia, but it did not find evidence of objective or quantitative improvement in sleep.[34] Melatonin, on the other hand, has been associated with small but significant improvements in sleep latency, sleep efficiency, and total sleep duration.[35]

Benzodiazepine Receptor Agonists (BzRAs)

Most agents currently approved by the FDA for use in insomnia include drugs that act as BzRAs. The BzRAs for insomnia consist of older benzodiazepines and newer BzRAs that are structurally dissimilar to benzodiazepines. Benzodiazepine hypnotics (estazolam, flurazepam, quazepam, temazepam, and triazolam) and the newer BzRAs (eszopiclone, zaleplon, and zolpidem) all bind to the GABA type A receptor and facilitate transmission of negative chloride ions across nerve cell membranes, thus leading to hyperpolarization of the cell.

All of these hypnotic agents are effective in reducing latency to sleep onset, and those with longer half-lives may also decrease wakefulness during sleep and increase total sleep time.[23] Except for triazolam, benzodiazepines tend to have long half-lives, which may explain their greater tendency to produce sedation and cognitive and psychomotor impairment during the daytime. The newer BzRAs in general have shorter half-lives and are therefore less likely to produce next-day impairment. Those with particularly short half-lives, including zaleplon and zolpidem, are primarily useful for sleep-onset problems; zaleplon can even be dosed during the night if needed, except within 4 hours of the desired wake-up time, so it may be useful for patients who do not have difficulty falling asleep initially but waken during the night and have trouble falling back asleep. Eszopiclone and the modified-release formulation of zolpidem have longer durations of action and can aid sleep onset as well as sleep maintenance.

Common side effects for BzRAs (both benzodiazepines and newer BzRAs) include sedation, cognitive impairment, and motor incoordination/ataxia. Abrupt discontinuation may produce rebound insomnia. These agents all have potential to lead to dependence or abuse in some individuals, and thus their use should be avoided in individuals with a history of substance abuse. Benzodiazepines should not be used in patients with obstructive sleep apnea, since they can exacerbate apnea through relaxation of the upper airway muscles as well as increase the arousal threshold. An National Institutes of Health (NIH) consensus panel concluded that adverse events are probably more severe with the use of benzodiazepines than with newer BzRAs.[2]

Hypnotics have also been associated with infrequent but potentially serious side effects such as severe allergic reactions or complex sleep-related behaviors; these have included parasomnia-like behaviors such as driving, eating, and engaging in sexual activity during the sleep period without fully awakening. Taking hypnotics at higher-than-recommended dosages or combining them with other sedatives or alcohol is more likely to produce these adverse events.

Ramelteon

Ramelteon, the first non-BzRA approved by the FDA for treatment of insomnia, acts as an agonist at type 1 and 2 melatonin receptors in the brain, although it is structurally dissimilar to melatonin. Ramelteon has a short half-life and has been shown to decrease latency to sleep onset, but it does not consistently increase total sleep time; it is indicated for use in sleep-onset insomnia. Ramelteon is not classified as a controlled substance and has not been shown to have abuse potential, cause next-day impairment, or lead to withdrawal or rebound insomnia.[36] Potentially serious side effects are similar to those reported for BzRAs; rare cases of severe allergic reactions (angioedema of the tongue and upper airway) as well as amnesia and complex sleep-related behaviors have been reported with use of ramelteon. Ramelteon should not be combined with fluvoxamine because this leads to dramatic increases in ramelteon blood levels.

Sedating Antidepressants

Other agents that are frequently used to treat insomnia include sedating antidepressants, anticonvulsants, and antipsychotics, although there are relatively few data for any of these agents regarding use for insomnia and they are generally not approved by the FDA for this indication. An important exception is the recent FDA approval of low-dose doxepin for sleep-maintenance insomnia. Sedating antidepressants include trazodone, mirtazapine, and tricyclic agents such as doxepin and amitriptyline. When prescribed for insomnia, they are generally used in dosages that are much lower than those generally indicated for the treatment of depression. If they are to be used as a single agent to treat both insomnia and depression, they should be prescribed at a therapeutic dose, although frequently they are used in low doses in combination with first-line agents such as selective serotonin reuptake inhibitors (SSRIs) in patients with depression. The sedating antidepressants in general act via antagonism of histamine, alpha-1, and serotonin type 2 (5HT2) receptors.

There is some limited evidence to suggest that trazodone can reduce sleep latency and increase sleep time.[37] Side effects include hangover sedation, gastrointestinal distress, blurred vision, dizziness, and headache. Cardiovascular effects, although infrequent, include orthostatic hypotension and arrhythmia. Trazodone-induced priapism is a medical emergency.

In addition to their sleep-promoting effects, tricyclic antidepressants (TCAs) tend to suppress REM sleep, which can lead to REM sleep rebound and insomnia upon abrupt withdrawal. They can also exacerbate restless legs and periodic limb movements, and precipitate REM sleep behavior disorder in susceptible individuals. Other side effects include next-day hangover, anticholinergic effects (e.g., dry mouth, orthostatic hypotension, constipation), cardiotoxicity (prolongation of QT interval and high lethality in overdose), and weight gain.

Recent studies, however, have demonstrated that very low doses of doxepin (up to 6 mg) can improve sleep efficiency and increase sleep duration in adults and elderly patients with primary insomnia[38,39] without leading to significant anticholinergic side effects or hangover. At these low doses, doxepin is presumed to act through binding to histamine (H1) receptors. The FDA recently approved low-dose doxepin for treatment of sleep-maintenance insomnia; it is not a controlled substance and at these low doses does not appear to lead to tolerance, withdrawal, amnesia, or complex sleep-related behaviors, in contrast to other approved hypnotics.

Mirtazapine has lower toxicity and fewer side effects than the TCAs, but weight gain is common. Other side effects include daytime sedation and dizziness. Studies in patients with major depression have shown improvements in subjective and objective sleep measures.[40]

All antidepressants have the potential to cause mania in patients with underlying bipolar disorder and may increase suicidal ideation in some individuals, so patients should be monitored carefully. They may also induce or exacerbate restless legs syndrome and REM sleep behavior disorder.[41] In general, there are insufficient data to support the use of sedating antidepressants (other than doxepin) as first-line treatment for primary insomnia, but they may be useful in patients with comorbid depression or in patients who should not take BzRAs.

Anticonvulsants

Although they are not approved by the FDA for treatment of insomnia, several anticonvulsants have been shown to have sleep-inducing properties, including gabapentin and pregabalin, which have been reported to decrease pain and improve sleep in fibromyalgia patients.[42] They are structural analogues of GABA and act on voltage-gated calcium channels to decrease release of excitatory neurotransmitters. Both have been reported to increase slow-wave sleep, but there are relatively few data regarding their efficacy in insomnia. Tiagabine also has been shown to increase slow-wave sleep and may improve sleep continuity,[43] likely through inhibition of GABA reuptake. Side effects of these agents include daytime sedation, dizziness, and cognitive impairment; gabapentin and pregabalin can also produce weight gain. There is evidence of benefit of these agents to patients with insomnia related to pain conditions, including fibromyalgia, since they also may decrease pain levels.

Antipsychotics

Several of the newer atypical antipsychotic medications, notably quetiapine and olanzapine, have increasingly been used for insomnia, although these agents are not approved by the FDA for the treatment of insomnia. Although their primary mechanism of action is to block dopamine type 2 (D2) receptors, they also block histamine and 5HT2C receptors. Limited studies have demonstrated improved sleep efficiency and increased total sleep with these agents, [44,45] but they have potentially serious side effects that limit their utility in patients who do not have other indications for their use, such as psychotic or bipolar disorders. Side effects include daytime sedation, weight gain, metabolic syndrome, lipid abnormalities, tardive dyskinesia, and increased mortality in elderly patients. They can also exacerbate restless legs and produce akathisia that can worsen sleep problems.

Choosing a medication

The choice of an agent should be guided by factors such as clinical symptoms, treatment goals, response to previous treatment, comorbid conditions, and pharmacology of all other medications used by the patient.[46] Issues such as patient preference and cost also need to be taken into account. Pharmacotherapy approaches recommended by the AASM for patients with primary insomnia are listed in Table 3.9, and information on specific agents is listed in Table 3.10.

Table 3.9 Pharmacotherapy for Insomnia[23]

Treatment Recommendations

1. Short/intermediate-acting BzRA or ramelteon. Choose based on patient factors.
2. Alternative BzRA or ramelteon. Choose based on response to previous choice.
3. Sedating low-dose antidepressant (AD).* May be useful for patients with depression, treatment failures, or those for whom BzRAs are contraindicated.
4. Combination of BzRA and AD.* May minimize toxicity by using two agents at lower doses.

Not Recommended

1. Other prescription drugs (e.g., gabapentin, tiagabine, quetiapine, olanzapine).* These agents are **not** currently recommended due to insufficient evidence for efficacy for insomnia, but they may be helpful for sleep in patients with other disorders for which they are indicated (e.g., anticonvulsants in chronic pain conditions or atypical antipsychotics for psychiatric disorders).
2. Over-the-counter agents (e.g., antihistamines, valerian, melatonin).* Potential side effects, limited efficacy data.
3. Other agents (barbiturates, chloral hydrate, meprobamate, methaqualone, propofol).* These agents should not be used for insomnia due to toxicity and risk for abuse and dependence.

* Not approved by the U.S. FDA for the treatment of insomnia.

Source: Schutte-Rodin S, Broch L, Buysse D, et al. Clinical guideline for the evaluation and management of chronic insomnia in adults. *J Clin Sleep Med.* 2008 Oct 15;4(5):487–504.

Table 3.10 Pharmacological Treatment for Insomnia

Drug	Dose Range (mg)	Dose in Elderly (mg)	Half-life (h)	Peak plasma level (h after admin)	FDA Indication	Side Effects
Benzodiazepine Receptor Agonists: Benzodiazepines						
Estazolam	1–2	0.5	10–24	2	I: SO, SM	
Flurazepam	15–30	15	47–100	2	I: SO, SM	
Quazepam	7.5–15	7.5	25–41	1.5	I: SO, SM	Dizziness, drowsiness, lightheadedness, ataxia, amnesia, GI symptoms
Temazepam	7.5–30	7.5	6–16	1	I	
Triazolam	0.25–0.50	0.125–0.250	1.5–5.5	2	I	
Benzodiazepine Receptor Agonists: Nonbenzodiazepines						
Eszopiclone	2–3	1–2	5–6	1	I: SO, SM	Unpleasant taste, dry mouth, dizziness, drowsiness, amnesia, GI symptoms
Zaleplon	10–20	5–10	1	1	I: SO	Dizziness, headache, GI symptoms, drowsiness, amnesia
Zolpidem	10	5	2.6 (5 MG), 2.5 (10 MG)	1.6	I: SO	
Zolpidem extended release	6.25–12.5	6.25	2.8	1.5	I: SO, SM	
Melatonin Receptor Agonist						
Ramelteon	8	8	1–2.6	0.75	I: SO	Drowsiness, dizziness, interaction with fluvoxamine

Antidepressants*

Amitriptyline	50–100	20	10–28 (including the metabolite nortriptyline)	4–8	MDD	Drowsiness, dizziness, confusion, blurred vision, dry mouth, constipation, urinary retention, arrhythmias, orthostatic hypotension, weight gain, exacerbation of restless legs, periodic limb movements, or REM-sleep behavior disorder
Doxepin	75–100	25–50	8–24	2–3	I: SM; MDD (higher doses)	
Mirtazapine	15–45	7.5–15	20–40	2	MDD	Drowsiness, dizziness, increased appetite, constipation, weight gain
Trazodone	50–400	25–150	7	1	MDD	Drowsiness, dizziness, headache, blurred vision, dry mouth, arrhythmias, orthostatic hypotension, priapism

Anticonvulsants*

Clonazepam	0.25–0.50	0.25	30–40	1–4	Anxiety, seizures	Drowsiness, dizziness, ataxia, depression, nervousness, reduced intellectual ability
Gabapentin	300–600	300	5–7	2–4	Seizures, neuralgia	Drowsiness, dizziness, emotional lability, ataxia, tremor, blurred vision, diplopia, nystagmus, myalgia, peripheral edema, weight gain
Pregabalin	50–300	50	6.3	1.5	Neuropathic pain, seizures, fibromyalgia	
Tiagabine	4–8	4	7–9	0.75	Seizures	Drowsiness, dizziness, ataxia, tremor, new-onset seizures in patients without epilepsy, difficulty in concentration or attention, nervousness, asthenia, abdominal pain, diarrhea, nausea

(continued)

Table 3.10 (continued)

Drug	Dose Range (mg)	Dose in Elderly (mg)	Half-life (h)	Peak plasma level (h after admin)	FDA Indication	Side Effects
Antipsychotics*						
Olanzapine	5–10	5	21–54	6	Schizophrenia. bipolar disorder	Drowsiness, dizziness, tremor, agitation, asthenia. extrapyramidal symptoms, dry mouth, dyspepsia, constipation, orthostatic hypotension, weight gain, new-onset diabetes mellitus
Quetiapine	25–200	25	6	1.5		
Risperidone	1–3	0.5–1.5	20–24	1		

* Not approved for treatment of insomnia by the U.S. Food and Drug Administration

I, insomnia; SO, sleep onset; SM, sleep maintenance; MDD, major depressive disorder.

In general, either a short- or intermediate-acting BzRA (zaleplon, zolpidem, eszopiclone, triazolam, or temazepam) or ramelteon should be used as the first-line agent, with the initial choice guided by the main symptoms (sleep onset and/or sleep maintenance difficulties). If the initial choice either produces undesirable side effects or is ineffective, another agent within this group should be selected based on the response to the first medication (e.g., if the first choice produces hangover, the second choice should be a drug with a shorter half-life). The lowest effective dose should be used to minimize side effects. In some patients, intermittent dosing regimens, such as 2 out of every 3 nights or up to 3 to 5 nights per week, may be sufficient, particularly if insomnia is not a nightly occurrence. However, those with severe, chronic conditions may require nightly dosing.

Some agents with sleep-inducing properties should not be used because of their potential for severe adverse events, their low toxic-to-therapeutic ratio, and risk for dependence. These include barbiturates, meprobamate, chloral hydrate, and anesthetic agents such as propofol.

The duration of pharmacotherapy for insomnia depends on the clinical situation. Although some patients may not require more than several weeks of treatment, many may require more chronic therapy. Newer agents such as eszopiclone, extended-release zolpidem, ramelteon, and low-dose doxepin do not have FDA labeling that limits duration of treatment, and placebo-controlled studies have shown continued efficacy for up to 6 months for some of these agents. In general, patients should be reassessed within 1 month of starting a medication for insomnia and monitored at least once every 6 months on chronic treatment to document continued efficacy and to assess for potential side effects, development of tolerance, and escalation of dose.

Terminating treatment with hypnotics may lead to rebound insomnia, which may be even more severe than the insomnia prior to treatment. For patients taking BzRAs, particularly at higher doses, there is also the potential for withdrawal. If sleeping medications are to be discontinued, they should be tapered gradually, with dose reductions made not more frequently than several days apart. Intermittent dosing may also be helpful as part of a tapering schedule. Use of adjunctive cognitive and behavioral therapies has also been demonstrated to improve success rates in hypnotic discontinuation.

When to Refer to a Sleep Specialist

Patients who fail to respond to the treatment recommendations outlined above and/or those who have symptoms suggestive of other primary sleep disorders such as sleep apnea or movement disorders may benefit from evaluation by a sleep specialist. Specialists in behavioral sleep medicine can provide cognitive behavior therapy and other therapies, but they may not be readily available in all areas. When insomnia is thought to be related to possible psychiatric illness, it is preferable to first refer the patient for psychiatric evaluation and treatment, then consider referral to a sleep specialist if the insomnia persists after the psychiatric issues have been addressed.

References

1. Ohayon MM, Roth T. Place of chronic insomnia in the course of depressive and anxiety disorders. *J Psychiatr Res.* 2003 Jan-Feb;37(1):9–15.

2. National Institutes of Health. National Institutes of Health State of the Science Conference statement on Manifestations and Management of Chronic Insomnia in Adults, June 13–15, 2005. *Sleep.* 2005 Sep 1;28(9):1049–57.

3. Roth T, Ancoli-Israel S. Daytime consequences and correlates of insomnia in the United States: results of the 1991 National Sleep Foundation Survey. II. *Sleep.* 1999;22 Suppl 2:S354–8.

4. Katz DA, McHorney CA. The relationship between insomnia and health-related quality of life in patients with chronic illness. *J Fam Pract.* 2002;51(3):229–35.

5. Suka M, Yoshida K, Sugimori H. Persistent insomnia is a predictor of hypertension in Japanese male workers. *J Occup Health.* 2003 Nov;45(6):344–50.

6. Ford DE, Kamerow DB. Epidemiologic study of sleep disturbance and psychiatric disorders: An opportunity for prevention? *JAMA.* 1989;262(11):1479–84.

7. Chang PP, Ford DE, Mead LA, et al. Insomnia in young men and subsequent depression. The Johns Hopkins Precursors Study. *Am J Epidemiol.* 1997 Jul 15;146(2):105–14.

8. Ohayon MM, Roth T. What are the contributing factors for insomnia in the general population? *J Psychosom Res.* 2001 Dec;51(6):745–55.

9. Ishigooka J, Suzuki M, Isawa S, et al. Epidemiological study on sleep habits and insomnia of new outpatients visiting general hospitals in Japan. *Psychiatry Clin Neurosci.* 1999;53(4):515–22.

10. Ohayon MM. Epidemiology of insomnia: what we know and what we still need to learn. *Sleep Med Rev.* 2002 Apr;6(2):97–111.

11. Peterson MJ, Benca RM. Sleep in mood disorders. *Psychiatr Clin North Am.* 2006 Dec;29(4):1009–32; abstract ix.

12. Manber R, Edinger JD, Gress JL, et al. Cognitive behavioral therapy for insomnia enhances depression outcome in patients with comorbid major depressive disorder and insomnia. *Sleep.* 2008 Apr 1;31(4):489–95.

13. Fava M, McCall WV, Krystal A, et al. Eszopiclone co-administered with fluoxetine in patients with insomnia coexisting with major depressive disorder. *Biol Psychiatry.* 2006 Mar 30.

14. Bonnet MH, Arand DL. Hyperarousal and insomnia: state of the science. *Sleep Med Rev.* 2010 Feb;14(1):9–15.

15. Riemann D, Spiegelhalder K, Feige B, et al. The hyperarousal model of insomnia: a review of the concept and its evidence. *Sleep Med Rev.* 2010 Feb;14(1):19–31.

16. Riemann D, Kloepfer C, Berger M. Functional and structural brain alterations in insomnia: implications for pathophysiology. *Eur J Neurosci.* 2009 May;29(9):1754–60.

17. Spielman AJ, Caruso LS, Glovinsky PB. A behavioral perspective on insomnia treatment. *Psychiatric Clin North Am.* 1987;10(4):541–54.

18. Lichstein KL, Durrence HH, Taylor DJ, et al. Quantitative criteria for insomnia. *Behav Res Ther.* 2003 Apr;41(4):427–45.

19. Buysse DJ, Reynolds CF, 3d, Monk TH, et al. The Pittsburgh Sleep Quality Index: a new instrument for psychiatric practice and research. *Psychiatry Res.* 1989;28(2):193–213.

20. Bastien CH, Vallieres A, Morin CM. Validation of the Insomnia Severity Index as an outcome measure for insomnia research. *Sleep Med.* 2001 Jul;2(4):297–307.

21. Johns MW. A new method for measuring daytime sleepiness: the Epworth Sleepiness Scale. *Sleep.* 1991 Dec;14(6):540–5.

22. Krupp LB, LaRocca NG, Muir-Nash J, et al. The Fatigue Severity Scale. Application to patients with multiple sclerosis and systemic lupus erythematosus. *Arch Neurol.* 1989 Oct;46(10):1121–3.

23. Schutte-Rodin S, Broch L, Buysse D, et al. Clinical guideline for the evaluation and management of chronic insomnia in adults. *J Clin Sleep Med.* 2008 Oct 15;4(5):487–504.

24. American Academy of Sleep Medicine. *International Classification of Sleep Disorders: Diagnostic and Coding Manual,* 2nd ed. Westchester, IL: American Academy of Sleep Medicine, 2005.

25. Krell SB, Kapur VK. Insomnia complaints in patients evaluated for obstructive sleep apnea. *Sleep Breath.* 2005 Sep;9(3):104–10.

26. Ebben MR, Spielman AJ. Non-pharmacological treatments for insomnia. *J Behav Med.* 2009 Jun;32(3):244–54.

27. Bootzin R, Epstein D, Wood JM. Stimulus control instructions. In: Hauri PJ, ed. *Case Studies in Insomnia.* New York: Plenum Press, 1991:19–28.

28. Spielman AJ, Saskin P, Thorpy MJ. Treatment of chronic insomnia by restriction of time in bed. *Sleep.* 1987;10(1):45–56.

29. Morin CM, Bootzin RR, Buysse DJ, et al. Psychological and behavioral treatment of insomnia: update of the recent evidence (1998–2004). *Sleep.* 2006 Nov 1;29(11):1398–414.

30. Smith MT, Perlis ML, Park A, et al. Comparative meta-analysis of pharmacotherapy and behavior therapy for persistent insomnia. *Am J Psychiatry.* 2002;159(1):5–11.

31. Morgenthaler T, Kramer M, Alessi C, et al. Practice parameters for the psychological and behavioral treatment of insomnia: an update. An American Academy of Sleep Medicine report. *Sleep.* 2006 Nov 1;29(11):1415–9.

32. Drugs for insomnia. *Treat Guidel Med Lett.* 2009 Mar;7(79):23–6.

33. Richardson GS, Roehrs TA, Rosenthal L, et al. Tolerance to daytime sedative effects of H1 antihistamines. *J Clin Psychopharmacol.* 2002 Oct;22(5):511–5.

34. Fernandez-San-Martin MI, Masa-Font R, Palacios-Soler L, etal. Effectiveness of valerian on insomnia: a meta-analysis of randomized placebo-controlled trials. *Sleep Med.* 2010 Jun;11(6):505–11.

35. Brzezinski A, Vangel MG, Wurtman RJ, et al. Effects of exogenous melatonin on sleep: a meta-analysis. *Sleep Med Rev.* 2005 Feb;9(1):41–50.

36. Zammit G. Comparative tolerability of newer agents for insomnia. *Drug Saf.* 2009;32(9):735–48.

37. Rosenberg RP. Sleep maintenance insomnia: strengths and weaknesses of current pharmacologic therapies. *Ann Clin Psychiatry.* 2006 Jan-Mar;18(1):49–56.

38. Roth T, Rogowski R, Hull S, et al. Efficacy and safety of doxepin 1 mg, 3 mg, and 6 mg in adults with primary insomnia. *Sleep.* 2007 Nov 1;30(11):1555–61.

39. Scharf M, Rogowski R, Hull S, et al. Efficacy and safety of doxepin 1 mg, 3 mg, and 6 mg in elderly patients with primary insomnia: a randomized, double-blind, placebo-controlled crossover study. *J Clin Psychiatry.* 2008 Oct;69(10):1557–64.

40. Shen J, Chung SA, Kayumov L, et al. Polysomnographic and symptomatological analyses of major depressive disorder patients treated with mirtazapine. *Can J Psychiatry*. 2006 Jan;51(1):27–34.

41. Wilson S, Argyropoulos S. Antidepressants and sleep: a qualitative review of the literature. *Drugs*. 2005;65(7):927–47.

42. Hauser W, Bernardy K, Uceyler N, Sommer C. Treatment of fibromyalgia syndrome with gabapentin and pregabalin—a meta-analysis of randomized controlled trials. *Pain*. 2009 Sep;145(1–2):69–81.

43. Walsh JK, Zammit G, Schweitzer PK, et al. Tiagabine enhances slow wave sleep and sleep maintenance in primary insomnia. *Sleep Med*. 2006 Mar;7(2):155–61.

44. Sharpley AL, Vassallo CM, Cowen PJ. Olanzapine increases slow-wave sleep: evidence for blockade of central 5-HT(2C) receptors in vivo. *Biol Psychiatry*. 2000 Mar 1;47(5):468–70.

45. Wine JN, Sanda C, Caballero J. Effects of quetiapine on sleep in nonpsychiatric and psychiatric conditions. *Ann Pharmacother*. 2009 Apr;43(4):707–13.

46. Krystal AD. A compendium of placebo-controlled trials of the risks/benefits of pharmacological treatments for insomnia: the empirical basis for U.S. clinical practice. *Sleep Med Rev*. 2009 Aug;13(4):265–74.

Chapter 4

Sleep Apnea and Related Disorders

The major sleep-related breathing disorders are obstructive sleep apnea (OSA) and central sleep apnea (CSA). OSA is characterized by an airway obstruction despite continued effort to breathe. CSA, which is far less common, involves cessation of both respiratory effort and airflow. Both result in inadequate ventilation during sleep, and patients often present with daytime symptoms of excessive sleepiness and/or insomnia. Snoring is a common problem that often signifies the presence of OSA. Sleep-related breathing disorders can occur in children as well as adults, although they are more common in adults.

Snoring

Description

Snoring refers to loud breathing sounds during sleep that are produced by vibrations of upper airway structures. It occurs more commonly during inspiration but can also occur during expiration, and it is more frequent in NREM than in REM sleep. Snoring can be as loud as 70 decibels in severe cases.[1]

Epidemiology

Snoring occurs regularly in about one third of adults and is more common in men than women.[2,3] The prevalence is increased in the obese and with age; at least half of middle-aged and older adults snore habitually. As discussed below, loud and/or frequent snoring may indicate the presence of sleep apnea. Snoring appears to be associated with daytime sleepiness independently of OSA.[4]

Pathophysiology

Snoring results from the vibration of soft tissues in the upper airway, including the uvula, soft palate, and pharyngeal walls. Any factors that decrease upper airway muscle tone during sleep, such as use of alcohol or sedative-hypnotic medications, can worsen snoring. Smoking as well as exposure to secondhand smoke is associated with increased snoring prevalence, presumably through irritation and inflammation of the upper airway. Other factors that reduce flow through the upper airway, such as nasal congestion, enlarged tonsils and/or adenoids, and sleeping in the supine position, can also lead to increased snoring. Medical factors such as obesity, hypothyroidism, and acromegaly, as well as craniofacial abnormalities such as retrognathia or micrognathia, can increase the risk of snoring.

Evaluation and Diagnosis

Snoring can range from a benign condition to an indication of a serious sleep disorder. Often it is a nuisance to the bed partner, who may have difficulty sleeping due to the noise. The diagnosis is clinical, based on report of the patient and/or bed partner.

Clinical evaluation should include the frequency of snoring, estimation of loudness, and factors that make it worse, such as use of alcohol, tobacco, sedative medications or sleeping in the supine position. Physical factors that may contribute to snoring, such as obesity, enlarged neck circumference, and upper airway compromise, should be evaluated. Evaluation of the upper airway should include examination for enlarged tonsils and airway size; the Mallampati classification is frequently used, and those with higher scores are more likely to have sleep apnea[5] (Fig. 4.1). Referral to an otolaryngologist for more definitive assessment of the upper airway should be considered for individuals seeking treatment for simple snoring with possible upper airway compromise.

Patients should also be screened for hypertension and hypothyroidism. Because snoring can signify the presence of sleep apnea, all patients with significant snoring should be screened for possible apnea (see next section). The recommended evaluation procedure is described in Table 4.1.

Treatment

In many cases, snoring can be treated with interventions that improve patency of the upper airway; these include weight loss, avoidance of supine sleep, and elimination of factors such as alcohol or sedative use at bedtime (Table 4.2). Other nonsurgical options include measures to enhance nasal airflow such as nasal dilators and use of mandibular-advancing oral appliances or tongue-retaining devices; an appropriately trained dentist or orthodontist generally fits these. Although continuous positive airway pressure (CPAP) is effective in eliminating snoring, it is generally not covered by insurance for this purpose alone.

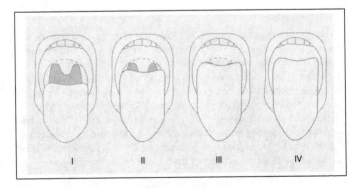

Figure 4.1 Mallampati classification diagrams

Table 4.1 Evaluation of Snoring and OSA

Clinical history (preferably obtained with bed partner present)
1. Snoring frequency and loudness
2. Effect of sleeping position (supine vs. nonsupine)
3. Presence of allergies, nasal congestion; use of tobacco, alcohol, sedative or hypnotic medications
4. Symptoms of sleep apnea: awakening with a sense of choking or gasping, witnessed apneas, daytime sleepiness (others listed in Table 4.3)

Physical examination
1. BMI and blood pressure
2. Neck circumference (>43 cm/17 in for men or >41 cm/16 in for women indicates increased risk for sleep apnea)
3. Upper airway for deviated septum, nasal obstruction, enlarged tonsils/adenoids, enlarged tongue, crowded pharynx, retrognathia, micrognathia
4. Cardiovascular and pulmonary systems

Laboratory testing if indicated
1. Thyroid function
2. Insulin growth factor 1 or growth hormone level if acromegaly suspected

Table 4.2 Treatment of Simple Snoring

Lifestyle changes
1. Weight loss
2. Avoid supine sleep. This can be accomplished through various devices that can be worn to prevent sleeping on the back.
3. Avoid use of alcohol.
4. Stop smoking, including eliminating exposure to secondhand smoke.

Nonsurgical treatments
1. Decrease or eliminate use of sedating medications, particularly at bedtime.
2. Use of nasal decongestants (nasal steroids) if congestion is present
3. Oral appliances (mandibular advancement or tongue-retaining)
4. Nasal dilators
5. Continuous positive airway pressure (CPAP); usually not covered by insurance for simple snoring

Surgical treatments (indicated for treatment of anatomic pathology)
1. Removal of nasal polyps
2. Correction of deviated nasal septum
3. Tonsillectomy, adenoidectomy
4. Uvulopalatopharyngoplasty and laser-assisted uvulopalatoplasty
5. Radiofrequency treatment of turbinates, soft palate, and tongue base

Surgical options should generally be reserved for those with significant structural abnormalities of the upper airway (e.g., enlarged tonsils or adenoids, deviated septum, craniofacial deformities). Surgery for idiopathic snoring has not been demonstrated to be particularly successful, and randomized, controlled trials for surgical treatments are generally lacking.[6] Nevertheless, patients are often interested in surgical treatments because of the hope for an immediate cure. The more commonly used surgical approaches include uvulopalatopharyngoplasty, laser-assisted uvulopalatoplasty, and radiofrequency ablation.

When to Refer to a Sleep Specialist

Patients with snoring and daytime symptoms suggesting possible sleep apnea should be referred for further evaluation including sleep laboratory testing.

Obstructive Sleep Apnea

Description

OSA is a common cause of sleep disruption resulting in daytime sleepiness. It is characterized by repeated episodes of partial to complete collapse of the upper airway during sleep that occur despite continuing efforts to breathe and result in episodes of decreased ventilation lasting at least 10 seconds. These events can occur up to 50 or more times per hour in severe cases and cause intermittent reductions in oxyhemoglobin saturation and increases in carbon dioxide levels. The obstructive events are generally terminated by brief arousals that restore airway patency but also lead to sleep fragmentation and daytime sleepiness. OSA is strongly predictive of hypertension, cardiovascular disease, stroke, diabetes, impaired cognitive function, hypersomnolence, decrements in daytime function, and premature all-cause and cardiovascular morbidity.[7] Treatment of apnea appears to reverse these risks.

The most common symptoms of OSA are loud snoring, witnessed apneas, and excessive daytime sleepiness. Snoring is often associated with snorting or gasping sounds at the end of the respiratory event. Although the vast majority of individuals with OSA (up to 95%) report snoring, it is important to remember that not all snorers have clinically significant apnea. Patients with apnea can also experience episodes of waking up with a sensation of choking or gasping for air. Bed partners often report witnessing episodes of apnea, and this is a frequent cause for individuals to come in for assessment for possible OSA. Daytime sleepiness is also found in the majority of patients with sleep apnea, but it is not strictly correlated with the severity of the apnea. Like snoring, daytime sleepiness is also seen in a variety of other conditions, so is not specific to OSA.

Other associated symptoms of OSA can include nighttime symptoms such as sweating, nocturia, gastroesophageal reflux, impotence, waking with a dry mouth, and insomnia or restless sleep. Daytime sequelae include morning headaches; cognitive impairment that may manifest itself in problems with attention and concentration; and changes in mood, including depression, anxiety, and irritability. Common clinical features of OSA are listed in Table 4.3.

Table 4.3 Symptoms of OSA
Nighttime symptoms
• Snoring
• Waking up choking or gasping for air
• Witnessed apneas
• Disrupted sleep/insomnia
• Nocturia
• Diaphoresis at night
Daytime symptoms
• Daytime sleepiness or fatigue
• Morning headaches
• Dry mouth upon awakening
• Problems with memory, concentration, performance
• Mood or personality changes

Epidemiology

In the United States, an estimated 17% of adults have at least mild sleep apnea (characterized by five or more apnea and/or hypopnea events per hour of sleep) and about 6% of adults have apnea that is moderate to severe (at least 15 events per hour of sleep).[8] Apnea is about two to three times more prevalent in men than women, but the prevalence of apnea in women increases after menopause. Two of the most significant risk factors for OSA in both men and women are age and weight. The prevalence of apnea is at least doubled in adults age 50 to 69 compared to those age 30 to 49 and is also strongly correlated with BMI: being overweight (BMI > 25) probably accounts for about 60% of cases of OSA. Given the rising obesity rates in the United States, it is likely that the prevalence of OSA will also continue to increase.

Other risk factors include craniofacial or upper airway anatomic features that can predispose even normal-weight individuals to have OSA, such as enlarged tonsils and adenoids, retrognathia, enlarged tongue, and enlarged soft palate.[9] The association of OSA with these characteristics likely accounts for the increased incidence of apnea in some families and possibly in certain racial groups; for example, apnea may be more severe in Asians in relation to BMI. Increased rates of apnea are seen in a range of medical conditions, particularly hypothyroidism, polycystic ovary syndrome, and pregnancy, and in association with medication or substance use. Risk factors are listed in Table 4.4.

OSA is also associated with an increased prevalence of cardiovascular disease, cerebrovascular disease, and type 2 diabetes.[7, 10] Given that the risk factors for these disorders overlap with the risk factors for OSA, causal relationships are difficult to ascertain. However, untreated apnea is associated with an increased risk of developing hypertension and increased mortality from cardiovascular causes, whereas treatment of apnea appears to decrease these risks, suggesting a contributory role of OSA for cardiovascular disease.

Table 4.4 Risk Factors for OSA
• Male gender
• Menopause
• Increasing age
• BMI > 25
• Increased neck circumference (>43 cm in men or >41 cm in women)
• Family history of OSA
• Craniofacial or upper airway features that predispose to obstruction
• Smoking, including secondhand smoke
• Alcohol use
• Medications
• Anesthetics
• Barbiturates
• Benzodiazepines
• Growth hormone
• Narcotics
• Testosterone
• Medical conditions
• Acromegaly
• Depression
• Diabetes mellitus
• Down syndrome
• Hypertension
• Hypothyroidism
• Neuromuscular disorders
• Polycystic ovary syndrome
• Pregnancy
• Renal failure
• Stroke

Pathophysiology

Various factors contribute to the collapse of the upper airway during sleep.[9,11] Much of the upper airway above the level of the larynx is a flexible tube, particularly between the hard palate and larynx. It is therefore subject to collapse when negative intrathoracic pressure generated by attempts to breathe overcomes the forces that keep the upper airway open. During waking, activity of the upper airway dilator muscles, particularly the genioglossus, ensures that the airway remains open during inspiration. However, the generalized decrease of muscle tone during the transition into sleep leads to an increased tendency for airway collapse during inspiration, particularly in individuals with any additional factors that decrease the diameter of the upper airway or decrease dilator muscle activity. REM sleep is often associated with the most frequent or prolonged obstructions, possibly because of the generalized muscle atonia and decreased chemoreceptor sensitivity to changes in pCO_2 and pO_2. In slow-wave sleep, usually apnea is less severe and upper airway muscle activity is increased. Sleeping supine can worsen apnea, as gravity allows the tongue and related soft tissues to fall back towards the posterior wall of the pharynx, decreasing airway diameter. Genetic factors that lead to increased rates of apnea in some families have not yet been identified but could include genes that influence anatomy of the upper airway, obesity, and/or respiratory control.

The obstructive respiratory event is terminated by an arousal, likely as a result of hypoxia- and hypercapnia-induced increases in breathing effort leading to increased pleural pressure. The arousal, often lasting only a few seconds, is sufficient to increase the activity of the upper airway dilator muscles and stimulate respiration. Oxyhemoglobin saturation level usually returns to baseline, and when sleep resumes, the cycle of obstruction can repeat.

Evaluation

The majority of patients with clinically significant OSA are undiagnosed and untreated. Recognition of the signs and symptoms of potential OSA, particularly in primary care settings, is key to identifying those at risk. The clinical history should include screening those with clinical risk factors (see Table 4.4) regarding the symptoms of apnea (see Table 4.3). Useful screening tools include the Berlin Questionnaire (Appendix 4), which has been demonstrated to have good sensitivity in identifying individuals at risk for OSA, and the Epworth Sleepiness Scale[12] (Appendix 5). The Berlin includes three categories of symptoms; those who are positive in at least two of the categories are considered high risk for having OSA. Although the Epworth is not specific for apnea, and apnea severity is not always correlated with degree of perceived sleepiness, the scale is useful to identify patients with excessive sleepiness who may require further screening for sleep apnea or other causes of sleepiness. It can also be helpful to follow treatment response in apnea patients.

As in the case of snoring, physical examination should include at a minimum BMI, blood pressure, neck circumference, assessment of the upper airway, and cardiovascular and pulmonary examination. Patients with suspected apnea should have thyroid function testing and other tests as suggested by features of their history or physical examination.

Patients with suspected apnea should then be referred for sleep testing. A sleep medicine specialist can determine whether in-laboratory or portable (home) testing is appropriate and should meet with the patient for a consultation to discuss test results and make treatment recommendations.

Diagnosis

Although clinical history and examination can indicate which patients may be at higher risk for OSA, diagnosis requires polysomnographic testing in a sleep laboratory or unattended monitoring in the home setting (portable monitoring), provided by a sleep laboratory and interpreted by a sleep medicine specialist. Attended, full-channel polysomnography (PSG) (described in Chapter 2) has been the standard for diagnosis of OSA and is the preferred method because it is more comprehensive in assessing respiratory parameters as well as monitoring sleep patterns, apnea-related sleep disruption, electrocardiogram, limb movements, and patient behavior. However, given the high prevalence of OSA and the high cost of and limited access to in-laboratory PSG, less extensive home monitoring may be used as well. In 2007, the American Academy of Sleep Medicine released guidelines for the use of portable monitoring[13] (described in Chapter 2) for OSA. They recommended that portable (home) monitoring may be used in patients with a high probability of at least moderately severe OSA and without significant comorbid medical conditions or other suspected sleep disorders; portable monitoring can detect sleep-disordered breathing but generally does not record EEG or limb movements, so it cannot reliably detect other sleep disorders. As with attended monitoring, portable monitoring should be used in patients who have undergone appropriate and comprehensive clinical evaluation. In 2008, the U.S. Centers for Medicare and Medicaid Services approved portable monitoring for diagnosis of OSA and prescription of positive airway pressure therapies.

OSA is diagnosed when sleep testing indicates the presence of a sufficient number of obstructive respiratory events that occur during sleep (see Chapter 2). These events are defined as **obstructive apneas** if there is complete cessation of nasal and oral airflow for at least 10 seconds accompanied by continued breathing effort. **Hypopneas** are less severe cessations in breathing and are defined as at least a 30% reduction in airflow or effort (defined by thoracoabdominal excursion) and accompanied by at least a 4% drop in oxyhemoglobin desaturation. A **respiratory event-related arousal (RERA)** refers to a reduction in airflow that does not meet the criteria for a hypopnea or apnea but produces an arousal in the EEG. The **apnea–hypopnea index (AHI)** refers to the number of apneas and hypopneas that occur per hour of sleep. The AHI is usually calculated for the entire night of sleep, but it may also be separately calculated for supine versus non-supine sleep and/or NREM versus REM sleep. The **respiratory disturbance index (RDI)** refers to the number of apneas, hypopneas, and RERAs per hour of sleep.

The overall AHI is commonly used to determine the severity of OSA. In general, an AHI below 5 is not considered abnormal, more than 5 and less than 15 is considered mild OSA, 15 to 30 is considered moderate OSA, and over 30 is considered severe OSA. These categories are somewhat arbitrary and do not take into account factors such as degree of hypoxemia or frequency of arousals by respiratory events that may be too mild to be considered an apnea or hypopnea. However, epidemiologic studies suggest that patients with an AHI of 15 or greater are at increased risk for cardiovascular and all-cause mortality if their apnea remains untreated.

Treatment

Patients with OSA may be followed by sleep medicine specialists for ongoing treatment. A number of patients may require management for their OSA from their primary care providers, however, such as those with relatively straightforward conditions who respond well to treatment, or in cases where sleep medicine specialists may not be available to patients due to geographical or insurance-related factors.

The "gold standard" treatment for sleep apnea is positive airway pressure (PAP) therapy. It is the recommended standard of therapy for patients with moderate to severe OSA (AHI of 15 or greater)[14] but should also be strongly considered for those with an AHI between 5 and 15 and symptoms of daytime sleepiness or associated comorbidities such as hypertension, arrhythmia, or history of cardiac ischemia or stroke. Studies suggest that treatment of OSA with PAP decreases the rate of adverse cardiovascular events.[7]

PAP works by acting as a pneumatic splint to keep the upper airway open during sleep. It is usually titrated in the sleep laboratory during overnight PSG to ensure determination of the appropriate pressure that will eliminate respiratory events and snoring, either during a full-night titration study or a split-night study, where titration of CPAP is performed during the second half of the night after significant OSA has been identified.[14] Ideally, this should include demonstration of effectiveness during supine REM sleep, when apnea and related hypoxemia is often most severe. Titration may also be performed in the home setting, with autotitrating equipment in adult patients without severe hypoxemia or complex medical issues.[15]

Continuous positive airway pressure (CPAP) is the most common form of PAP therapy and is effective in most patients with OSA. Pressures of CPAP needed to eliminate OSA usually range from a low of 5 cm H_2O pressure to a high up to 24 cm H_2O pressure; not surprisingly, higher pressures are more difficult for many patients to tolerate. **Bilevel positive airway pressure (BPAP)** delivers two pressure settings, a higher one during inspiration, when collapse of the airway is most likely, and a lower one during expiration. It is sometimes better tolerated in patients who require high pressures to maintain airway patency; in those with hypoventilation such as with obesity hypoventilation syndrome or chronic obstructive pulmonary disease; and in those with a component of CSA. BPAP can also assist with ventilation. CPAP can also be used in an autotitrating setting **(autotitrating positive airway pressure [APAP])** that adjusts the pressure based on the breathing patterns and thus delivers a mean lower pressure across the night. APAP can also be used in the home setting in some cases to determine the CPAP pressure needed. APAP is also useful for making PAP more tolerable for patients who need high pressures only intermittently during the night, such as during REM sleep. However, APAP should not be used in patients with certain comorbidities, including heart failure, chronic obstructive pulmonary disease, obesity hypoventilation syndrome, and daytime or nocturnal hypoxemia; in these cases, APAP may worsen CSA or fail to maintain adequate ventilation. A sleep specialist is trained to determine the optimal mode of PAP therapy for each patient.

PAP therapy can reverse many of the symptoms of OSA. Benefits may include improving sleep quality, eliminating snoring, and decreasing daytime sleepiness. PAP use can also decrease many of the health risks associated with OSA, such as hypertension, arrhythmias, and mortality, particularly from cardiovascular and cerebrovascular events. Unfortunately, many patients with OSA fail to comply with PAP treatment; only about half of patients use it consistently.

Because compliance rates are low, increasing compliance with PAP therapy is one of the most important issues in the treatment of OSA.[16] It is critical to educate patients on the health benefits of PAP therapy and the risks of untreated apnea to improve compliance with treatment.[14] Patient education about the use of PAP therapy and the importance and benefits of OSA treatment, as well as early intervention to alleviate difficulties with usage, have been shown to improve compliance. Problems with compliance usually occur early in treatment, and compliance within the first week is predictive of long-term use. Newer equipment has monitoring software built in that can indicate the hours of nightly use, continued apnea, and mask leak. In general, the greater the perceived benefit of PAP to the patient, the better the compliance. Not surprisingly, those with more severe symptoms, particularly daytime sleepiness, are more likely to use PAP, whereas those with mild OSA are often less compliant.

More common side effects to PAP therapy include mask leaks, leaking air through the mouth, swallowing air resulting in abdominal distention, and nasal congestion, rhinorrhea, nosebleeds, or dryness of nasal and oral passages. Mask leaks can produce irritation or dryness of the eyes. Some individuals feel claustrophobic wearing the mask or find it uncomfortable; sometimes it can cause skin irritation or sores. More serious side effects are very rare, but instances of trauma from high air pressure such as pneumothorax, rupture of tympanic membranes, and pneumocephalus have been reported. Some of the common problems that patients encounter with PAP therapy are listed in Table 4.5.

Patients receiving PAP therapy need to clean their equipment regularly. They also should have their masks replaced at regular intervals and their machines checked to ensure adequate pressure delivery; the durable medical equipment provider who supplied the PAP equipment usually does this. Masks should be fitted by respiratory therapists, PSG technologists, or other trained professionals.

Oral appliances, including those that advance the mandible or tongue-retaining devices, may be helpful in patients with mild to moderate apnea who do not wish to use PAP therapy or those with supine-dependent apnea.[17] These devices are generally better tolerated than PAP therapy but are less effective. To assess the treatment response, a sleep study, either at home or in the sleep laboratory, should be performed. Side effects include jaw, temporomandibular joint or tooth pain, dry mouth, or changes in the bite. Oral appliances should be fitted by a trained professional, usually a dentist or orthodontist. Mandibular advancement devices should not be used in patients with poor or missing dentition or in those with CSA.

Patients with mild to moderate apnea may benefit from use of a small valve inserted into the nares and affixed with adhesive that creates positive airway

Table 4.5 Problems Leading to Decreased Compliance with PAP Therapy and Suggested Solutions
Nasal congestion, rhinorrhea, sneezing, epistaxis
This can be worsened by mouth leak. Try adding heated humidification to the PAP unit or nasal saline irrigation and/or nasal corticosteroids.
Mouth leak
Add chin strap to PAP headgear or use full face mask that covers nose and mouth.
Mask leak
May present with eye irritation or conjunctivitis. Ensure that mask is properly fitting and that straps are not too tight or too loose.
Difficulty exhaling
Add C-flex, a temporary reduction of pressure at the beginning of exhalation. Consider use of autotitrating PAP or bilevel PAP.
Aerophagia
Elevate head of bed.
Change to BPAP; consider APAP.
Difficulty falling asleep while wearing PAP
Gradually acclimate/desensitize patient to wearing PAP.
Consider trial of hypnotic, but avoid medications that can worsen apnea such as benzodiazepines.
Use ramp setting on PAP machine that starts the patient on a lower pressure at the beginning of the night and gradually increases pressure, presumably after patient has fallen asleep.
Pressure sores, skin breakdown
Cover pressure points with moleskin or chamois cloth.
Alternate use of different types of masks (e.g., nasal mask and nasal pillows).
Claustrophobia from wearing mask
Use desensitization procedures, including gradual accommodation to the mask and pressure.
Use nasal pillow mask.

pressure during expiration (EPAP).[18] The nasal EPAP device may be better tolerated than CPAP for some patients and reduces AHI in some patients. For patients with significant apnea treated with either oral appliances or nasal EPAP devices, follow-up sleep studies (either in-laboratory or unattended home studies) should be performed to document treatment efficacy.

For patients whose apnea is mild or moderate and occurs only during supine sleep, avoiding the supine sleeping position may be adequate.[19] There are a number of commercial products available that can be worn to prevent patients from rolling over onto their backs during sleep. Alternatively, patients can try wearing a fanny pack with tennis balls, or wear a homemade device consisting of a T-shirt with a pocket sewn down the middle of the back that can hold three or four tennis balls.

Surgical treatments for apnea,[20] as for snoring (see above), are indicated in some individuals with clearly defined anatomic problems that may be contributing to obstruction, such as enlarged tonsils or adenoids, or nasal polyps.[21] In these cases, surgery may help to decrease the severity of OSA or possibly eliminate the need for additional treatment. Other surgical approaches may include elimination of excessive tissue in the upper airway (e.g., uvulopalatopharyngoplasty) or increasing the dimensions of the upper airway (e.g., mandibular advancement). The efficacy of these procedures is debatable, and patients may require multiple procedures before clinical improvement is evident. However, they may be a recourse for patients who cannot tolerate or are unsuccessfully treated with noninvasive modalities. In any case, patients who undergo surgery for moderate to severe OSA should undergo sleep testing after surgery to assess efficacy.

One highly effective surgical approach that is used for patients with severe OSA is tracheostomy; this is usually reserved for life-threatening cases who cannot tolerate PAP therapy, severely obese patients who have hypoventilation not correctable with PAP therapy, or those with upper airway obstructions that cannot be overcome by PAP. The tracheostomy can be plugged during the day and is opened for sleeping.

The only potentially curative treatment for OSA is weight loss, in cases where apnea is caused by obesity. Even moderate weight loss can reduce the severity of apnea.[19] Weight loss, however, can be quite challenging for the severely obese. Bariatric surgery has been shown to reduce the severity of OSA or eliminate the need for PAP therapy in the majority of morbidly obese patients. After a loss of about 10% of body weight, patients on PAP therapy should be reassessed in terms of apnea severity and level of PAP needed.

All patients with OSA should be assessed for factors that may be contributing to apnea severity. Medications and substances that may contribute to upper airway muscle relaxation or increase arousal threshold should be eliminated if possible (see Table 4.4). Nasal congestion should be treated, including through the use of saline rinses, fluticasone nasal spray, or other topical nasal corticosteroid.[19] Patients should be advised to avoid sleep deprivation and supine sleep, as these can worsen apnea severity. Most importantly, patients should be counseled regarding the hazards of drowsy driving; those with severe daytime sleepiness who have not responded to therapy or are not compliant should not operate motor vehicles.

Some patients continue to experience daytime sleepiness despite treatment of OSA and resolution of apneic events in sleep. Assuming full compliance and demonstrated effectiveness of therapy, a variety of factors may contribute to this and should be assessed, including other sleep disorders, insufficient sleep, medication effects, and mood disorders; these should be treated if present. In patients with persistent sleepiness despite elimination of other potential causes, modafinil has been shown to improve daytime alertness and has been recommended as a treatment standard for OSA patients with daytime sleepiness despite PAP treatment.[19] Armodafinil may also be used to treat sleepiness associated with sleep apnea. See chapter 5 for further information about use of modafinil and armodafinil for sleepiness. Note that stimulants are not a substitute for correcting the nocturnal airway obstruction in OSA and should not be used as a primary treatment for apnea.

Therapies for OSA are listed in Table 4.6.

When to Refer to a Sleep Specialist

Patients in whom OSA is suspected should be sent to a sleep medicine specialist for diagnosis, including sleep testing. The specialist will determine

---

Table 4.6 Therapies for OSA

A. Lifestyle changes

1. Weight loss. Reassess severity of apnea with sleep testing after 10% loss of body weight.

2. Avoid supine sleep. This can be accomplished through various devices that can be worn to prevent sleeping on the back.

3. Avoid use of alcohol.

4. Stop smoking, including eliminating exposure to secondhand smoke.

B. Nonsurgical treatments

1. Positive airway pressure (either CPAP or BPAP); standard of care for moderate to severe OSA, patients with any degree of OSA and daytime sleepiness

2. Oral appliances (mandibular advancement or tongue-retaining); these are options for mild or moderate OSA in patients who cannot tolerate PAP, particularly those whose apnea is worse while supine. They may be used in patients who have continued apnea following upper airway surgery. Note that mandibular advancement devices cannot be used in patients with inadequate dentition to hold the device.

   a. Appliance should be fitted by a dental specialist and patient should have regular follow-up with this specialist.

   b. Sleep testing should be performed with the oral appliance to verify resolution/improvement of apnea.

3. Nasal EPAP device

4. Adjunctive measures

   a. Decrease or eliminate use of sedating medications, particularly at bedtime.

   b. Treat nasal congestion with topical steroids or saline rinses.

C. Surgical treatments

1. Surgical treatment is indicated for treatment of specific, surgically correctable pathology deemed responsible for the OSA. Examples include:

   a. Removal of nasal polyps

   b. Correction of deviated nasal septum

   c. Tonsillectomy, adenoidectomy

2. Other treatments that may be considered when noninvasive treatments fail or are refused include procedures such as uvulopalatopharyngoplasty, laser-assisted uvulopalatoplasty, maxillomandibular advancement osteotomy, radiofrequency ablation.

3. Patients require repeat sleep study after surgical treatments (best performed at least 6 weeks after surgery) since response is not consistent and additional treatment, including PAP therapy, may be needed.

4. Tracheostomy is effective and may be considered when other treatments fail or are refused.

whether an in-laboratory test or portable home test is appropriate, based on the clinical situation, and in most cases will perform at least a consultation and initiate the appropriate therapy. Referral back to a sleep medicine specialist should be considered when symptoms that were present before treatment return of snoring while using PAP therapy, gain or loss of more than 10% of body weight, development of cardiac disease (particularly congestive heart failure or arrhythmia), or development of cerebrovascular disease.

Central Sleep Apnea

Description

CSA is characterized by apneas in sleep that occur not as a result of obstruction, but rather due to a lack of breathing effort. Central apneas consist of cessation of airflow lasting at least 10 seconds unaccompanied by any ventilatory effort. CSA is far less common than OSA and tends to occur in those with congestive heart failure, neurological disorders, and stroke. It is also more common in patients taking opioid narcotics and is exacerbated at high altitude. Prevalence is increased in men and the elderly. CSA can also emerge as a side effect of PAP therapy in OSA; in this case it is referred to as complex apnea.

Although CSA shares with OSA some similar clinical features, such as excessive daytime sleepiness, morning headaches, and frequent nocturnal awakenings, patients with CSA may be asymptomatic. Furthermore, unlike OSA patients, snoring, if present, is usually mild, and patients may be normal weight to obese. Daytime symptoms may be absent, but if present are similar to those seen in OSA, including daytime sleepiness and cognitive impairment. Common symptoms are listed in Table 4.7.

Epidemiology

Epidemiological data regarding CSA prevalence is variable, with reported prevalences ranging from a few percent to over 50%, depending on the population studied and the definition of central apnea used.[7,22] Occasional central

Table 4.7 Symptoms of CSA
Nighttime symptoms
• Waking up with shortness of breath or gasping for air
• Witnessed apneas
• Restless sleep/insomnia
• Snoring absent or mild
Daytime symptoms
• Daytime sleepiness or fatigue (may be absent)
• Morning headaches
• Problems with memory, concentration, or performance
• Mood or personality changes

apneas during sleep may be fairly common in the population and not necessarily pathological.

A number of risk factors have been associated with increased rates of CSA (Table 4.8), including male gender, increasing age, and various medical disorders, including diabetes, stroke, heart failure, and neuromuscular disorder. Chronic opioid use can also contribute to CSA.[23]

Pathophysiology

During sleep, ventilation is largely regulated by arterial PCO_2 ($PaCO_2$); if it drops below the threshold value needed to stimulate respiration, an apnea will occur. Individuals with idiopathic or primary central apnea have an increased ventilatory response to CO_2. This in turn decreases $PaCO_2$ during waking and sleep below the threshold needed to produce ventilation in sleep, resulting in sleep-related apneas. Changes in the metabolic control of respiration at transitions into sleep also contribute to central apneas that may occur only at sleep onset and then disappear as the sleep state becomes stable and persistent.

A minority of patients with central apnea may have diminished sensitivity to CO_2. They hypoventilate during wakefulness and even more so during sleep, particularly REM sleep. These include some severely obese individuals with **obesity hypoventilation syndrome**, which is characterized by hypercapnia during waking; during sleep, hypercapnia may worsen and they often show prolonged decreases in baseline oxygen saturation not related to apneas or hypopneas. Obesity hypoventilation syndrome can occur in conjunction with OSA or CSA but can also occur alone in the absence of significant apnea. Patients with this disorder may have excessive daytime sleepiness, erythrocytosis from their chronic hypoxemia, and even right heart failure and edema in severe cases.

Heart failure patients may display Cheyne-Stokes respiration during both wakefulness and sleep, caused by the effects of increased circulation time on metabolic control of breathing. This pattern is characterized by a gradual,

Table 4.8 Risk Factors for CSA
• Male gender
• Menopause
• Increasing age
• Living at higher altitude
• Nasal obstruction
• Medications
• Benzodiazepines
• Opioids
• Medical conditions
• Diabetes mellitus
• Heart failure
• Stroke
• Neuromuscular disorders

waxing-and-waning pattern of airflow and respiratory effort, whereas patients with idiopathic CSA show more abrupt cessation and initiation of breathing.

Evaluation and Diagnosis

Further evaluation for apnea should be considered for patients with risk factors and symptoms. Given the overlap in presentation between OSA and CSA, the general evaluation process should be similar.

Overnight PSG is required for diagnosis of CSA. Respiratory effort monitoring is critical for distinguishing central from obstructive events, and can be difficult. Furthermore, many patients exhibit both central and obstructive events (mixed apnea syndrome). Esophageal balloon monitors are the most sensitive but are more difficult to use and not always well tolerated by patients. Measuring CO_2 levels with transcutaneous or end-tidal monitors may be helpful in detecting hypercarbic patients. Portable monitoring is not recommended for patients who are suspected of having CSA.[13]

A diagnosis of CSA requires that the patient have more than five central apneas per hour of sleep, each lasting at least 10 seconds. In addition, the patient must have at least one associated symptom of daytime sleepiness, insomnia or disturbed sleep, or waking short of breath. In patients with both CSA and OSA, the majority of the events should be central to make a primary diagnosis of CSA; for research purposes, thresholds are often higher.

Treatment

PAP therapy has been shown to be helpful in treating CSA including Cheyne-Stokes breathing.[7,22] Some patients may respond to standard CPAP, but others may require pressure cycled ventilation, such as BPAP or **adaptive servoventilation (ASV).** ASV delivers variable pressure that maintains minute ventilation below the threshold that can lead to hypocapnia and periodic breathing and thus may be useful in a range of conditions that exhibit central apneas, including primary central apnea, Cheyne-Stokes respiration, complex sleep apnea (central apnea that develops in response to CPAP), and apnea and ataxic breathing in patients on chronic opioids. Unfortunately, it is not yet clear whether PAP treatment of central apnea in heart failure patients reduces mortality, although studies using ASV suggest that it might lead to better outcomes in this population than CPAP.[24,25]

Other treatment options include supplemental oxygen therapy, which may help to prevent hypoxemia and reduces hypocapnia in patients with increased sensitivity to CO_2. It can cause further increases in $PaCO_2$ in already hypercarbic patients, however, so should be used with caution.

A variety of medications may be helpful to increase respiratory drive during sleep, although they are not FDA approved for these uses.[24] Acetazolamide, which increases respiratory drive by producing metabolic acidosis, has been used most widely, and appears to reduce central apneas, but most studies have been short-term. Other medications that have been administered to central apnea patients include theophylline and medroxyprogesterone. There are relatively few data on the use of any of these agents on central apnea, and they all have potentially significant side effects that limit their use.

In patients without significant hypoxemia and in whom central apneas appear to be related to severe sleep fragmentation, hypnotics may help to consolidate sleep and stabilize breathing.

Recommended CSA treatment is described in Table 4.9.

When to Refer to a Sleep Specialist

Patients with CSA should be referred to sleep specialists for testing and management.

A summary of the sleep-related breathing disorders discussed in this chapter can be found in Table 4.10.

Table 4.9 Treatment of CSA

1. Treat any underlying medical problems such as heart failure, pulmonary disease.
2. Weight loss for obese patients
3. Eliminate medications that may be contributing to apnea (e.g., opioids).
4. Trial of PAP therapy (CPAP, BPAP, adaptive servoventilation)
5. Supplemental oxygen
6. Pharmacotherapy with respiratory stimulants (acetazolamide, medroxyprogesterone, theophylline, clomipramine, naloxone)
7. Use of hypnotic to consolidate sleep if apneas are primarily seen at transition into sleep

---

Table 4.10 Sleep-Related Breathing Disorders[26]

A. Primary central sleep apnea

1. At least one of the following:
   a. Excessive daytime sleepiness
   b. Frequent arousals or insomnia
   c. Awakening short of breath
2. Polysomnography demonstrates at least five central apneas per hour of sleep.

B. Cheyne-Stokes breathing pattern

1. Polysomnography demonstrates at least 10 central apneas and hypopneas per hour of sleep with crescendo–decrescendo pattern of tidal volume, leading to arousals and fragmentation of sleep.
2. Breathing disorder is associated with a serious medical disorder (heart failure, stroke, renal failure).

C. High-altitude periodic breathing

1. Recent ascent to at least 4,000 meters
2. Polysomnography demonstrates at least 5 central apneas per hour in a periodic breathing pattern with cycle length of 12–34 seconds.

D. Central apnea due to drug or substance

1. Regular use of opioid for at least 2 months
2. Polysomnography shows one of the following:
   a. At least five central apneas per hour of sleep
   b. Periodic breathing with at least 10 central apneas and hypopneas per hour with crescendo–decrescendo pattern of tidal volume, leading to arousals and fragmentation of sleep

(continued)

Table 4.10 (continued)

E. Primary sleep apnea of infancy

1. Apnea of prematurity

   a. Central apneas at least 20 seconds in duration or shorter-duration events (may include obstructive events) accompanied by physiologic compromise (decreased heart rate, hypoxemia, other symptoms)

   b. Occurs in infants <37 weeks conceptual age

2. Apnea of infancy

   a. Central apneas at least 20 seconds in duration or shorter-duration events (may include obstructive events) accompanied by physiologic compromise (bradycardia, cyanosis, pallor, hypotonia)

   b. Occurs in infants at least 37 weeks conceptual age

F. Obstructive sleep apnea, adult

1. At least one of the following:

   a. Daytime sleepiness, sleep attacks, unrefreshing sleep, fatigue, insomnia

   b. Waking up gasping or choking

   c. Bed partner reports snoring and/or apneas

AND

2. Polysomnography shows the following:

   a. At least five respiratory events (apneas, hypopneas, or respiratory-related arousals) per hour of sleep

   b. Evidence of respiratory effort during at least part of each respiratory event

OR

3. Polysomnography shows the following:

   a. At least 15 respiratory events per hour of sleep

   b. Evidence of respiratory effort during at least part of each respiratory event

G. Obstructive sleep apnea, pediatric

1. Caregiver reports snoring and/or labored, obstructive breathing and at least one of the following:

   a. Paradoxical inward movement of ribcage during inspiration

   b. Arousals with movement

   c. Diaphoresis

   d. Neck hyperextension in sleep

   e. Excessive daytime sleepiness, hyperactivity, or aggressive behavior

   f. Slowed growth

   g. Morning headache

   h. Secondary enuresis

2. Polysomnography demonstrates at least one respiratory event per hour of sleep (defined as apnea or hypopnea lasting at least two respiratory cycles) and at least one of the following:

   a. One of the following:

      i. Frequent arousals from sleep with increased respiratory effort

      ii. Arterial oxygen desaturation with apneas

      iii. Hypercapnia during sleep

      iv. Negative swings in esophageal pressure

Table 4.10 (continued)

b. Periods of hypercapnia and/or desaturation during sleep with snoring, paradoxical inward movement of ribcage during inspiration, and at least one of the following:

   i. Frequent arousals from sleep

   ii. Negative swings in esophageal pressure

H. Sleep-related nonobstructive alveolar hypoventilation, idiopathic

1. Polysomnography demonstrates episodes of shallow breathing lasting at least 10 seconds and associated with arterial oxygen desaturation and arousals from sleep, or brady-tachycardia.

I. Congenital central alveolar hypoventilation syndrome

1. Shallow breathing, or cyanosis and apnea occurs during perinatal period.

2. Hypoventilation worse during sleep

3. Absent or diminished rebreathing ventilatory response to hypoxia and hypercapnia

4. Polysomnography demonstrates severe hypercapnia and hypoxia, predominantly without apnea.

J. Sleep-related hypoxemia due to pulmonary parenchymal or vascular pathology

1. Hypoxemia due to lung or pulmonary vascular disease

2. Polysomnography demonstrates one of the following:

   a. SpO_2 during sleep is 5 min with nadir at no higher than 85%.

   b. SpO_2 is 30% of sleep time.

   c. $PaCO_2$ during sleep is significantly increased compared to waking or abnormally high, as determined by arterial blood gas.

K. Sleep-related hypoventilation/hypoxemia due to lower airways obstruction

1. Lower airways obstructive disease present (forced expiratory volume exhaled in 1 sec/forced vital capacity ratio <70% of predicted)

2. Polysomnography or sleeping arterial blood gas demonstrates one of the following:

   a. SpO_2 during sleep is 5 min with nadir at no higher than 85%.

   b. SpO_2 is 30% of sleep time.

   c. $PaCO_2$ during sleep is significantly increased compared to waking or abnormally high, as determined by arterial blood gas.

L. Sleep-related hypoventilation/hypoxemia due to neuromuscular and chest wall disorders

1. Neuromuscular or chest wall disorder present (e.g., amyotrophic lateral sclerosis, multiple sclerosis, obesity)

2. Polysomnography or sleeping arterial blood gas demonstrates one of the following:

   a. SpO_2 during sleep is 5 min with nadir at no higher than 85%.

   b. SpO_2 is 30% of sleep time.

   c. $PaCO_2$ during sleep is significantly increased compared to waking or abnormally high, as determined by arterial blood gas.

M. Sleep apnea/sleep-related breathing disorder, unspecified

1. Used to classify disorders of sleep-related breathing disorder that cannot be classified into any of the above categories

---

Adapted with permission from the American Academy of Sleep Medicine. *International Classification of Sleep Disorders: Diagnostic and Coding Manual*, 2nd ed. Darien, IL: American Academy of Sleep Medicine, 2005.

References

1. Wilson K, Stoohs RA, Mulrooney TF, et al. The snoring spectrum: acoustic assessment of snoring sound intensity in 1,139 individuals undergoing polysomnography. *Chest.* 1999 Mar;115(3):762–70.

2. Nieto FJ, Young TB, Lind BK, et al. Association of sleep-disordered breathing, sleep apnea, and hypertension in a large community-based study. Sleep Heart Health Study. *JAMA.* 2000 Apr 12;283(14):1829–36.

3. Ohayon MM, Guilleminault C, Priest RG, et al. Snoring and breathing pauses during sleep: telephone interview survey of a United Kingdom population sample. *BMJ.* 1997 Mar 22;314(7084):860–3.

4. Young T, Peppard PE, Gottlieb DJ. Epidemiology of obstructive sleep apnea: a population health perspective. *Am J Respir Crit Care Med.* 2002 May 1;165(9):1217–39.

5. Mallampati SR, Gatt SP, Gugino LD, et al. A clinical sign to predict difficult tracheal intubation: a prospective study. *Can Anaesth Soc J.* 1985 Jul;32(4):429–34.

6. Franklin KA, Anttila H, Axelsson S, et al. Effects and side-effects of surgery for snoring and obstructive sleep apnea—a systematic review. *Sleep.* 2009 Jan 1;32(1):27–36.

7. Somers V, White D, Amin R, et al. Sleep apnea and cardiovascular disease: an American Heart Association/American College of Cardiology Foundation scientific statement from the American Heart Association Council for High Blood Pressure Research Professional Education Committee, Council on Clinical Cardiology, Stroke Council, and Council on Cardiovascular Nursing Council. *J Am Coll Cardiol.* 2008;52:686–717.

8. Young T, Peppard PE, Taheri S. Excess weight and sleep-disordered breathing. *J Appl Physiol.* 2005 Oct;99(4):1592–9.

9. Punjabi NM. The epidemiology of adult obstructive sleep apnea. *Proc Am Thorac Soc.* 2008 Feb 15;5(2):136–43.

10. Tasali E, Mokhlesi B, Van Cauter E. Obstructive sleep apnea and type 2 diabetes: interacting epidemics. *Chest.* 2008 Feb;133(2):496–506.

11. Eckert DJ, Malhotra A. Pathophysiology of adult obstructive sleep apnea. *Proc Am Thorac Soc.* 2008 Feb 15;5(2):144–53.

12. Johns MW. A new method for measuring daytime sleepiness: the Epworth Sleepiness Scale. *Sleep.* 1991 Dec;14(6):540–5.

13. Collop NA, Anderson WM, Boehlecke B, et al. Clinical guidelines for the use of unattended portable monitors in the diagnosis of obstructive sleep apnea in adult patients. Portable Monitoring Task Force of the American Academy of Sleep Medicine. *J Clin Sleep Med.* 2007 Dec 15;3(7):737–47.

14. Kushida CA, Littner MR, Hirshkowitz M, et al. Practice parameters for the use of continuous and bilevel positive airway pressure devices to treat adult patients with sleep-related breathing disorders. *Sleep.* 2006 Mar 1;29(3):375–80.

15. Morgenthaler TI, Aurora RN, Brown T, et al. Practice parameters for the use of autotitrating continuous positive airway pressure devices for titrating pressures and treating adult patients with obstructive sleep apnea syndrome: an update for 2007. An American Academy of Sleep Medicine report. *Sleep.* 2008 Jan 1;31(1):141–7.

16. Weaver TE, Grunstein RR. Adherence to continuous positive airway pressure therapy: the challenge to effective treatment. *Proc Am Thorac Soc.* 2008 Feb 15;5(2):173–8.

17. Kushida CA, Morgenthaler TI, Littner MR, et al. Practice parameters for the treatment of snoring and obstructive sleep apnea with oral appliances: an update for 2005. *Sleep.* 2006 Feb 1;29(2):240–3.

18. Rosenthal L, Massie CA, Dolan DC, et al. A multicenter, prospective study of a novel nasal EPAP device in the treatment of obstructive sleep apnea: efficacy and 30-day adherence. *J Clin Sleep Med.* 2009 Dec 15;5(6):532–7.

19. Morgenthaler TI, Kapen S, Lee-Chiong T, et al. Practice parameters for the medical therapy of obstructive sleep apnea. *Sleep.* 2006 Aug 1;29(8):1031–5.

20. Aurora RN, Casey KR, Kriso D, et al. Practice parameters for the surgical modifications of the upper airway for obstructive sleep apnea in adults. *Sleep* 2010; 33(10):1408–13

21. Won CH, Li KK, Guilleminault C. Surgical treatment of obstructive sleep apnea: upper airway and maxillomandibular surgery. *Proc Am Thorac Soc.* 2008 Feb 15;5(2):193–9.

22. White DP. Central sleep apnea. In: Kryger M, Roth T, Dement W, eds. *Principles and Practice of Sleep Medicine*, 4th ed. Philadelphia: Elsevier Saunders, 2005:969–82.

23. Walker JM, Farney RJ, Rhondeau SM, et al. Chronic opioid use is a risk factor for the development of central sleep apnea and ataxic breathing. *J Clin Sleep Med.* 2007 Aug 15;3(5):455–61.

24. Bordier P. Sleep apnoea in patients with heart failure: Part II: Therapy. *Arch Cardiovasc Dis.* 2009 Oct;102(10):711–20.

25. Kasai T, Usui Y, Yoshioka T, et al. Effect of flow-triggered adaptive servo-ventilation compared with continuous positive airway pressure in chronic heart failure patients with coexisting obstructive sleep apnea and Cheyne-Stokes respiration. *Circ Heart Fail.* 2009 Nov 20.

26. American Academy of Sleep Medicine. *International Classification of Sleep Disorders: Diagnostic and Coding Manual*, 2nd ed. Westchester, IL: American Academy of Sleep Medicine, 2005.

Chapter 5

Excessive Sleepiness and Narcolepsy

Description

Excessive sleepiness is characterized by an increased tendency to fall asleep and/or the need to exert increased effort to stay awake in low-stimulus or inactive situations. When the condition is severe, sleep onset can occur in more active situations such as eating a meal or while in the midst of a conversation. Excessive sleepiness may also include the perception of needing too much sleep. Associated features often include problems with memory, concentration, and attention, as well as irritability.

Sleepiness should be distinguished from fatigue, which is a characterized by low energy or tiredness but is usually not associated with an increased tendency to fall asleep or an increased duration of total daily sleep. For example, many patients with chronic insomnia and an inability to fall asleep report fatigue, and may even spend extended periods of time in bed. Sleepiness is also distinct from stupor or other causes of decreased consciousness in that sleep will usually reverse the symptoms at least temporarily.

Epidemiology

Excessive sleepiness is a common symptom, and epidemiological studies suggest that about 5% of the population reports severe daytime sleepiness and up to 15% to 20% may have more moderate symptoms of feeling "usually sleepy during the daytime."[1] Sleeping "too much" is reported by up to about 5% of the population in several studies, although the definition of excessive sleep was not specified in most of these studies. A European study found that less than one third of those who report that they "sleep too much" reported obtaining more than 9 hours of sleep per day, however.[1]

Younger individuals are more likely to report increased quantity of sleep than older people, but there are not sufficient data regarding age-related effects on daytime sleepiness. There are not obvious gender-related differences in the prevalence of excessive sleepiness symptoms.

Complaints of excessive sleepiness, like insomnia, are highly correlated with psychiatric disorders, although not all of these individuals may have objective evidence of increased sleep amount or tendency. Almost half of individuals who reported hypersomnia in a general population study were found to meet criteria for a psychiatric disorder,[2] and the rates of lifetime history of psychiatric illness in young adults with hypersomnia tended to be even greater than in those with insomnia.[3] Conversely, individuals with mood disorders, in particular, have high rates of hypersomnia. Estimates for rates of hypersomnia vary considerably across studies but tend to range from about one quarter to three quarters of adults with mood disorders, with higher rates in younger adults and women; rates of hypersomnia appear to be lower in elderly depressed subjects.[4] Narcolepsy, one of the primary sleep disorders associated with excessive sleepiness, is relatively rare, and may affect up to 1 in 2,000 individuals in the U.S. population.[5]

Causes of Excessive Sleepiness

A variety of conditions can result in the complaint of excessive daytime sleepiness, including insufficient sleep, sleep disorders, medical and psychiatric disorders, and effects of medications or substances (Table 5.1). **Insufficient sleep**, defined as obtaining less sleep than needed, occurs in about 1 in 5 adults, although not all of these individuals report excessive sleepiness.[6,7] Typically, individuals with insufficient sleep will report obtaining amounts of sleep at night that are less than normal for their age group and will have increased amounts of sleep on weekends or during vacations (rebound or recovery sleep). Adolescents and young adults are more prone to insufficient sleep, and men more commonly restrict their sleep than women. Some individuals are naturally long sleepers, requiring 10 or more hours per night on a regular basis, and thus may be more susceptible to developing sleep restriction given the constraints of busy schedules.

A variety of **medical disorders** can contribute to excessive sleepiness. Neurological disorders, including head trauma, are commonly associated with increased sleepiness, likely because they affect systems that regulate sleep-wakefulness. Sleepiness may also be seen in a broad range of **psychiatric disorders**. Excessive sleepiness has been studied more in mood disorders than other psychiatric illnesses. Individuals with bipolar depression and a subset of those with major depression may complain of increased sleepiness rather than insomnia during depressive episodes. Seasonal affective disorder or winter depression also commonly presents with increased sleep duration and increased daytime sleepiness, primarily during the winter months, when the duration of daylight is reduced. The resolution or reduction of symptoms with light therapy supports the possibility that decreased light input to the central nervous system (CNS) may be partly responsible for triggering the episodes.

Many **medications and substances** can cause sedation, particularly those that increase gamma aminobutyric acid (GABA) release, are anticholinergic or antihistaminergic, or block 5HT-2 receptors. Substances of abuse such as alcohol and sedatives can cause sedation or sleepiness, and stimulants can result in increased sleepiness upon withdrawal.

Table 5.1 Common Causes of the Complaint of Excessive Sleepiness

Medical disorders
- Fibromyalgia and chronic fatigue syndrome
- Rheumatologic disorders
- Congestive heart failure
- Hypothyroidism
- Cancer

Neurological/degenerative disorders
- Head trauma
- Encephalitis
- Parkinson's disease
- Alzheimer's disease

Psychiatric disorders
- Mood disorders

Medications/substances
- Alcohol
- Anticonvulsants
- Antidepressants (mirtazapine, trazodone, tricyclics)
- Antipsychotics (clozapine, olanzapine in particular)
- Hypnotics
- Sedatives
- Withdrawal from stimulants

Sleep disorders
- Insufficient sleep/sleep deprivation
- Sleep apnea
- Sleep-related movement disorders
- Circadian rhythm disorders
- Narcolepsy
- Idiopathic hypersomnia
- Episodic hypersomnias (Kleine-Levin syndrome, menstrual-related hypersomnia)

Excessive sleepiness can occur in a number of primary sleep disorders. Those that cause sleep fragmentation at night such as **obstructive sleep apnea** (Chapter 4) and **sleep-related movement disorders** (Chapter 8) likely interfere with the normal homeostatic recovery that takes place during sleep. **Circadian rhythm disorders** (Chapter 6) produce sleepiness when an individual needs to be awake during the circadian phase that promotes sleep.

Other sleep disorders that cause hypersomnia include narcolepsy, idiopathic hypersomnia, and recurrent hypersomnia. The primary symptom of **narcolepsy** is excessive daytime sleepiness, which typically includes a chronic and persistent level of sleepiness, coupled with strong, sometimes irresistible urges to sleep that recur throughout the day.[5,8] These sleep attacks are more likely to occur during low-stimulus situations, such as while sitting, reading, watching television, and so forth. Narcoleptics often do not show increased total amounts of sleep across the day,[9] although increased sleep duration may occur in the early stages of the disorder.

Associated symptoms of narcolepsy may include cataplexy, sleep paralysis, and hypnagogic hallucinations; along with excessive daytime sleepiness, these symptoms form the narcolepsy tetrad. Excessive sleepiness is typically the first symptom to appear, with other symptoms sometimes occurring years later if at all.

The presence of cataplexy in a patient with excessive sleepiness is almost diagnostic of narcolepsy; it consists of a sudden loss of muscle tone, typically bilateral, that occurs suddenly in response to emotional stimuli. Most typically, cataplexy is triggered by laughter, but it can also occur with other strong emotions such as anger or surprise.[10] Cataplexy can be severe, resulting in the patient falling to the ground, but in many cases it is mild and is accompanied by symptoms such as the head nodding forward briefly, slight buckling at the knees, feeling suddenly weak or clumsy, or slurred speech. These attacks usually last seconds to minutes but can go on for much longer in rare cases. Narcolepsy is generally subdivided into forms with and without cataplexy.

Narcolepsy with cataplexy is thought to be caused by a loss of hypocretin-producing cells in the lateral hypothalamus.[11] Greater than 90% of individuals with cataplectic narcolepsy have significantly reduced levels of hypocretin in their cerebrospinal fluid, whereas reduced hypocretin levels occur in less than half of those with narcolepsy without cataplexy.

In narcolepsy, sleep paralysis and hallucinations may occur at sleep onset (hypnagogic) or upon awakening (hypnopompic); they frequently occur together. The paralysis affects all skeletal muscles except the extraocular muscles and the diaphragm, so patients are able to breathe and look around; this paralysis is identical to that which occurs during REM sleep. Similarly, narcolepsy-related hallucinations are more commonly visual but may be auditory or involve other dream experiences such as a sense of levitation.[10,12] Patients with narcolepsy also may suffer from nocturnal sleep problems such as insomnia due to fragmented sleep with frequent nocturnal arousals. They also have increased rates of other primary sleep disorders, including REM sleep behavior disorder, sleep-related movement disorders, and sleep apnea.

The strong association of the disorder with the human leukocyte antigen (HLA) DQB1*0602 suggests a possible autoimmune mechanism. At least 90% of narcoleptic patients with cataplexy express this HLA marker, but since it is relatively common in the general population, it is not diagnostically specific.[13] Narcolepsy can also occur secondary to CNS infections, head trauma, or tumors. Hypocretin levels have been reported to be low in some but not all of these cases.[14]

Idiopathic hypersomnia, like narcolepsy, is characterized by excessive daytime sleepiness, but without associated features of cataplexy, sleep paralysis, and hypnagogic hallucinations. It can occur with long sleep time (>10 hours per night) or in those with normal amounts of nighttime sleep. Episodic hypersomnias are characterized by intermittent periods of increased sleep duration and daytime sleepiness. **Kleine-Levin syndrome** tends to occur in adolescent boys and may be accompanied by symptoms of increased eating, cognitive dysfunction, hypersexuality, and/or aggressiveness. **Menstrual-related hypersomnia** occurs in women, usually in the days just prior to menses.

Evaluation of the Sleepy Patient

Patients with excessive daytime sleepiness should undergo evaluation similar to that described for insomnia (see Table 3.3), including obtaining a description of the sleep complaint, general sleep history, pertinent medical and psychiatric history, medication and substance use, and history of prior treatments. If substance abuse is suspected, a urine drug screen should be performed.

Specific features of the evaluation should include careful assessment of the sleep symptom(s). Does the patient sleep an insufficient, normal, or excessive amount per day? If daytime sleepiness is present, it needs to be distinguished from fatigue or decreased consciousness (e.g., stupor). Patients should be asked about associated symptoms of narcolepsy (cataplexy, sleep paralysis, and hypnagogic hallucinations) as well as a family history of narcolepsy or other sleep disorders.

Physical examination should document degree of alertness and the patient's behavior. Individuals with severe sleepiness may have difficulty staying awake during the examination; they can fall asleep in the reception area or examination room while waiting, or show signs of sleepiness such as yawning or stretching, increased rate of eye-blinking, ptosis or frank closure of the eyelids, or slurred speech. In the unusual case that a patient has an episode of cataplexy in front of a clinician, deep tendon reflexes should be tested; in cataplexy, they are absent.

Evaluation of excessive daytime sleepiness includes clinical evaluation of the subjective symptoms as well as use of validated questionnaires and sleep laboratory testing. Questionnaires may be used to assess subjective sleepiness and sleep patterns, as well as monitor response to therapy. The most commonly used questionnaire is the Epworth Sleepiness Scale (ESS; Appendix 5),[15] which was designed to measure the overall level of daytime sleepiness. It is an eight-item, self-rated scale that asks the subject to assess the likelihood of dozing or falling asleep in daily situations such as reading, watching TV, or riding as a passenger in an automobile. Each item is scored on a scale of 0 (no chance of dozing) to 3 (high chance of dozing), and the item scores are summed to yield a total score of 0 to 24. Significant daytime sleepiness is signified by scores above 10, whereas scores above 15 are thought to indicate severe sleepiness. ESS scores, however, are not always correlated with the degree of sleepiness measured on the Multiple Sleep Latency Test (MSLT).

Sleep diaries are useful to assess duration of sleep, pattern of sleep across the day, and tendency for daytime napping. They are particularly useful for detecting insufficient sleep or circadian rhythm disorders that may be contributing to the sleep complaints.

Sleep laboratory evaluation for excessive sleepiness should be performed in patients whose sleepiness is not obviously related to sleep deprivation or insufficient sleep, a medical or psychiatric disorder, or substance use or abuse. Testing may also be indicated in those whose sleepiness does not respond to treatment for the presumed cause. Sleep testing should include an overnight sleep study (polysomnography) to document the amount and kind of sleep obtained, as well as to assess for sleep disorders such as apnea or a sleep-related movement disorder that may be causing daytime sleepiness. If no obvious cause of daytime sleepiness is seen on polysomnography, the patient should undergo an MSLT the following day to determine the degree of daytime sleepiness.

The MSLT consists of four or five nap opportunities beginning 1.5 to 3 hours after waking up in the morning and repeated every 2 hours across the day (see Chapter 2). Patients are asked to lie in bed quietly and try to fall asleep; sleep onset is scored with the first epoch of any stage of sleep. Mean latencies of 8 minutes or less are suggestive of excessive sleepiness, but there can be a great deal of variability in both normal subjects as well as those with sleep disorders. Most patients with narcolepsy will show mean sleep latencies of less than 5 minutes. Note that the patient must have obtained a minimum of 6 hours of sleep the night prior to testing, and preferably the patient should have obtained the amount typically obtained on a normal night. If the patient is taking stimulant medications, they should be discontinued at least 2 weeks prior to the study. To detect sleep-onset REM periods (SOREMPs), REM sleep-suppressing medications such as antidepressants should also be discontinued if not clinically inadvisable; in the cases of long-acting agents such as fluoxetine, the washout period should be at least 4 weeks. Since it may take at least several days for an individual to recover from sleep restriction or deprivation, it is important that the MSLT or Maintenance of Wakefulness Test (MWT) is administered after a week of sufficient sleep, documented by a sleep diary.

The MWT determines the ability of an individual to stay awake under low-stimulus conditions and is sometimes used to determine response to treatment for daytime sleepiness (see Chapter 2); it is not indicated for making a diagnosis in a hypersomnic patient. In this test, the patient sits in a dimly lit, quiet room and is asked to sit still, look directly ahead, and try not to fall asleep.

If there is any suspicion of CNS pathology or lesion, appropriate brain imaging or clinical EEG studies should be performed. Low levels of hypocretin in the cerebrospinal fluid are highly suggestive of narcolepsy, with over 90% of narcoleptics with cataplexy showing low or undetectable levels. Patients with other disorders and associated sleepiness can also show reduced hypocretin levels, however, and hypocretin levels are not necessarily low in every narcoleptic.[16] There is currently no standard available clinical test for narcolepsy based on hypocretin measurement.

Diagnosis

An accurate diagnosis for the specific cause(s) of excessive sleepiness is necessary to determine the appropriate treatment, particularly since this may entail long-term use of stimulant medications. Table 5.2 provides guidelines for diagnosis of excessive sleepiness. Diagnostic criteria for hypersomnias of central origin are summarized in Table 5.3, and some of the key clinical features helpful for distinguishing disorders presenting with hypersomnia as a primary symptom are listed in Table 5.4. In general, objective testing of sleepiness with the MSLT is clinically indicated whenever narcolepsy or idiopathic hypersomnia is suspected, as well as in other situations when the tendency to fall asleep needs to be objectively verified.[17] However, interpretation of MSLT results is complicated by the fact that there are not well-established normative values, and results can be skewed by a number of factors and variables. Therefore, diagnosis should not rely solely on the results of the MSLT, but all available data need to be taken into consideration. If the MSLT results are inconsistent with other data, repeating the test may be useful. Nevertheless, a mean sleep latency of less than 8 minutes is considered consistent with excessive sleepiness. Similarly, a mean sleep latency of less than 8 minutes is considered abnormal on the MWT, although this test is more typically used to assess treatment response rather than for diagnosis.

In rare cases, a patient with excessive sleepiness and cataplexy witnessed by a clinician may be diagnosed with narcolepsy based on clinical presentation alone, but diagnosis of narcolepsy generally requires sleep laboratory testing. Sleep tendency is assessed on the MSLT, with narcoleptics typically showing an average sleep onset latency of less than 8 minutes across four or five naps, and the presence of at least two SOREMPs (a SOREMP is defined as REM sleep occurring with the 15-minute nap). The MSLT should occur after a night of

Table 5.2 Diagnosis of Excessive Sleepiness

A. Clinical history
1. Excessive daytime sleepiness
2. Increased or normal amounts of nocturnal sleep
3. Associated narcolepsy symptoms (cataplexy, sleep paralysis, hypnagogic hallucinations)
4. Sleep deprivation
5. Shift work

B. Comorbid illnesses
1. Medical disorders
2. Psychiatric disorders

C. Medications and substance use

D. Questionnaires (Epworth Sleepiness Scale)

E. Sleep log

F. Actigraphy (especially in cases where history or sleep log may be unreliable)

G. Polysomnography and MSLT (indicated for suspected narcolepsy, idiopathic hypersomnia, obstructive sleep apnea, sleep-related movement disorder)

H. MWT (may be used to assess ability to remain awake when this may need to be assessed for personal or public safety reasons; may be used to assess response to treatment)

Table 5.3 Hypersomnias of Central Origin[12]

Narcolepsy with cataplexy
- Excessive sleepiness lasting at least 3 months
- Presence of cataplexy, defined as sudden and transient loss of muscle tone, triggered by emotion
- Diagnosis confirmed by PSG followed by MSLT (mean sleep latency ≤8 minutes, 2 sleep onset REM periods); or hypocretin-1 level ≤110 pg/mL or ≤1/3 control value

Narcolepsy without cataplexy
- Excessive sleepiness lasting at least 3 months
- Typical cataplexy not present
- Diagnosis confirmed by PSG followed by MSLT (mean sleep latency ≤8 minutes, 2 sleep onset REM periods)

Narcolepsy due to medical condition
- Excessive sleepiness lasting at least 3 months
- Significant underlying medical condition accounts for sleepiness.
- Presence of one of the following:
- Cataplexy
- MSLT with mean sleep latency <8 minutes, 2 sleep onset REM periods
- Hypocretin-1 level ≤110 pg/mL or ≤1/3 control value

Recurrent hypersomnia (Kleine-Levin and menstrual-related hypersomnias)
- Recurrent episodes of sleepiness lasting 2 days to 4 weeks, occurring at least once per year
- Normal alertness, cognition, and behavior in between episodes

Idiopathic hypersomnia with long sleep time
- Excessive sleepiness lasting at least 3 months
- Difficulty waking up in the morning or from naps
- Documentation of prolonged sleep time (>10 hours) and short sleep latency on PSG
- MSLT shows mean sleep latency <8 minutes and <2 sleep onset REM periods.

Idiopathic hypersomnia without long sleep time
- Excessive sleepiness lasting at least 3 months
- Documentation of normal sleep time (6–10 hours)
- MSLT shows mean sleep latency <8 minutes and <2 sleep onset REM periods.

Behaviorally induced insufficient sleep syndrome
- Excessive sleepiness lasting at least 3 months
- Documentation that habitual sleep period is shorter than expected for age
- Sleep amount is significantly longer on weekends/vacations.
- PSG (if done) shows sleep latency <10 minutes, sleep efficiency >90%.
- MSLT (if done) shows mean sleep latency <8 minutes, with or without sleep onset REM periods.

Hypersomnia due to medical condition
- Excessive sleepiness lasting at least 3 months
- Medical or neurological disorder accounts for sleepiness.
- MSLT (if done) shows mean sleep latency <8 minutes and no more than one sleep onset REM period.

Table 5.3 (continued)

Hypersomnia due to drug or substance (abuse or medications)

• Excessive sleepiness

• Sleepiness due to current use, prior prolonged use, or recent discontinuation of drugs or a prescribed medication

Hypersomnia not due to substance or known physiological condition (nonorganic hypersomnia, NOS)

• Excessive sleepiness temporally associated with a psychiatric diagnosis

• PSG (if done) shows reduced sleep efficiency, increased number and duration of awakenings.

• MSLT (if done) results variable; may be normal.

Physiological (organic) hypersomnia, unspecified (organic hypersomnia, NOS)

• Excessive sleepiness lasting at least 3 months

• MSLT shows mean sleep latency <8 minutes and less than 2 sleep onset REM periods.

• Sleepiness thought to be due to physiological condition, but does not meet criteria for another diagnosis.

Source: American Academy of Sleep Medicine. *International Classification of Sleep Disorders: Diagnostic and Coding Manual*, 2nd ed. Westchester, IL: American Academy of Sleep Medicine, 2005.

Table 5.4 Sleep Disorders Associated with Excessive Sleepiness

Insufficient sleep syndrome

Clinical features: Daytime sleepiness associated with nocturnal sleep times that are significantly shorter than norms for age. Sleep is extended on weekends/holidays ("catch-up" sleep). More frequent in adolescents and young adults.

PSG: Short sleep latency, high sleep efficiency (>90%), increased sleep time when allowed to sleep ad libitum

MSLT: Mean sleep latency <8 minutes, often with presence of Stage 2 sleep

Long sleepers

Clinical features: Patients require extended amounts of sleep (usually >10 hours) per day, such that they appear to have insufficient sleep syndrome if they obtain significantly less sleep.

PSG: Increased sleep duration (at least 10 hours) when allowed to sleep ad libitum, even when not sleep-deprived

MSLT: Normal when not sleep-deprived

Narcolepsy

Clinical features: Sleepiness/sleep attacks; may have associated symptoms of cataplexy, sleep paralysis, and hypnagogic hallucinations. Nocturnal sleep may be fragmented. Increased incidence of REM sleep behavior disorder.

PSG: Short sleep latency (<10 minutes), reduced latency to REM sleep or sleep onset REM period (SOREMP), sleep fragmentation/frequent arousals

MSLT: At least 2 SOREMPs, mean sleep latency ≤8 minutes and usually <5 minutes.

Table 5.4 (Continued)

Idiopathic hypersomnia

Clinical features: Constant and severe daytime sleepiness with normal or increased (>10 hours) nocturnal sleep amount. May be associated with extreme difficulty awakening from sleep, including confusion upon awakening (sleep drunkenness).

PSG: Sleep efficiency normal to elevated (>85%)

MSLT: Mean sleep latency <8 minutes; <2 SOREMPs

Mood disorder

Clinical features: Daytime sleepiness or profound fatigue, usually worse during exacerbation of mood disorder. Nocturnal sleep time variable; time in bed may be extended.

PSG: Features may include reduced latency to REM sleep (<60 minutes), decreased slow-wave sleep, sleep fragmentation.

MSLT: Usually normal; may be decreased

Chronic fatigue syndrome/fibromyalgia

Clinical features: Debilitating fatigue, time in bed often increased, but sleep time not necessarily increased. Complaints of nonrestorative sleep.

PSG: Increased sleep latency, reduced sleep efficiency, reduced slow-wave sleep for age. Alpha intrusion may be present in NREM sleep.[33]

MSLT: Usually normal

Kleine-Levin syndrome

Clinical features: Episodes of increased sleep that may last days–weeks. Usually occurs in adolescents. Cognitive abnormalities, feeling of derealization, increased eating and weight gain, irritability, hypersexuality, depression may be present. Usually remits in <10 years.[34]

PSG: Increased daily sleep amount, decreased sleep efficiency; slowing of background EEG activity may occur.

MSLT: Unknown

---

polysomnography, as discussed above, to verify that no other primary sleep disorders may be producing the symptoms.

Treatment

Treatment depends on the underlying cause of the sleepiness. For individuals with insufficient sleep, careful attention to sleep hygiene and scheduling enough hours in bed is the most important intervention. Some individuals who may be naturally long sleepers may require a greater number of hours in bed than usual for their age group. Even in patients with sleep disorders that result in excessive sleepiness, such as narcolepsy, good sleep hygiene and avoidance of sleep deprivation are key components of treatment, since insufficient sleep can exacerbate symptoms. In general, stimulants should not be used as a substitute for obtaining needed sleep.

Medications or substances that may cause sedation should be discontinued if possible. Treatment of medical, psychiatric, or sleep disorders (e.g., apnea, movement disorders, and circadian rhythm disorders) that may be contributing to sleepiness should be optimized. However, in some cases sleepiness will persist even when the comorbid conditions are well controlled, and thus treatments targeted at the sleep complaint may be needed.

Behavioral strategies may be helpful for some patients. These include scheduled naps to decrease homeostatic pressure for sleep. Patients with narcolepsy, in particular, may benefit from short, strategic naps during the day. Alerting measures such as bright light, exercise, or sensory stimulation are usually only transiently effective and not adequate to prevent sleep in situations where alertness is critical, such as driving.[18]

In patients with hypersomnia not related to insufficient sleep, medication use, or psychiatric disorders, stimulant medications are indicated as a primary mode of therapy. Stimulants may also be considered for patients in whom sleepiness is persistent and clinically significant despite the above measures. Medications used for treating excessive sleepiness may include stimulants as well as other nonstimulants that may have alerting effects.

Caffeine, the stimulant most widely used by the world's population, is a methylxanthine that blocks adenosine receptors in the brain. It promotes wakefulness but tolerance can develop rapidly, resulting in withdrawal effects of increased sleepiness and headaches. Caffeine also can increase heart rate and blood pressure and it has a diuretic effect; in high doses it can cause palpitations, anxiety, agitation, gastrointestinal upset, and tremor. Although often used, sometimes in large amounts, by patients with excessive sleepiness, it is generally not sufficient as monotherapy for the treatment of hypersomnia disorders.

Stimulants indicated for the treatment of excessive sleepiness due to narcolepsy by the U.S. FDA include modafinil, methylphenidate, and amphetamines. In general, these drugs have been tested more extensively in patients with narcolepsy than with other disorders associated with excessive sleepiness, although they are likely helpful for treating hypersomnia associated with other conditions as well. Modafinil is recommended as first-line therapy for narcolepsy by the American Academy of Sleep Medicine because it is effective and has a better benefit-to-risk ratio than other stimulants;[19] it is listed as a Schedule IV substance by the FDA. Its enantiomer, armodafinil, has a similar half-life but different pharmacokinetic profile in that it produces a higher plasma concentration later in the day on a milligram-to-milligram basis.[20] Modafinil acts by blocking dopamine (DA) transporters and thus increasing extracellular DA levels in the brain.[21] Its main side effects include headache, dry mouth, insomnia, nausea, and anxiety.[22,23] Cardiovascular effects may also occur, such as hypertension, palpitations, or chest pain. Rare cases of dermatologic reactions and hypersensitivity, including Stevens-Johnson syndrome and toxic epidermal necrolysis, have also been reported.

Methylphenidate and amphetamines are also considered effective for treating excessive daytime sleepiness due to narcolepsy and may be effective for other causes of hypersomnia as well.[23] They are available in a variety of formulations, including immediate- and extended-release preparations. These medications improve alertness by increasing levels of monoamines, particularly norepinephrine (NE) and DA. Methylphenidate blocks reuptake of NE and DA, amphetamine in addition enhances release of NE and DA, and methamphetamine is more lipophilic than amphetamine, thus resulting in increased levels in the brain.[24,25] These drugs are all FDA Schedule II compounds because they are potentially addictive.[26,27] Side effects include insomnia, anorexia, headache, nausea, motor tics, tremor, and hypertension; they should be used with caution in patients with hypertension or cardiac disease. All stimulants can potentially lead to psychiatric complications such as anxiety, irritability, mania, and even psychosis.

Selegiline is an irreversible monoamine oxidase (MAO) inhibitor, selective for MAO B,[28] that may improve alertness and decrease cataplexy in narcolepsy.[29] It has the advantage of not being a scheduled substance, but its main disadvantages are that it requires a low-tyramine diet and can cause hypertensive crisis when used with other medications such as antidepressants or stimulants. Selegiline is not FDA approved for narcolepsy, however.

Stimulants are not always helpful for other symptoms of narcolepsy, including cataplexy, sleep paralysis, and hypnagogic hallucinations. Antidepressants were the mainstay of treatment for these symptoms until the introduction of sodium oxybate (FDA Schedule III), which is not only effective for the cataplexy but also decreases daytime sleepiness and nocturnal sleep fragmentation. Tricyclic antidepressants (TCAs) may be helpful through their suppression of REM sleep. The TCAs most commonly used in narcolepsy include protriptyline, desipramine, and imipramine. TCAs are not FDA approved for the treatment of narcolepsy. Antidepressants carry the black box warning of increased suicidal thinking and behavior in children and adolescents with major depressive disorder and other mood disorders. The use of TCAs is limited by their potentially significant side effects, including anticholinergic effects (blurred vision, urinary retention, orthostatic hypotension, constipation, dry mouth, and dizziness), decreased libido, weight gain, and cardiac conduction changes; this latter effect makes them particularly dangerous in overdose. TCAs can also have withdrawal effects such as rebound cataplexy.

Selective serotonin reuptake inhibitors (SSRIs; particularly fluoxetine), dual serotonin and NE reuptake inhibitors (SNRIs; e.g., venlafaxine), and NE reuptake inhibitors (e.g., duloxetine, reboxetine) have been shown to reduce cataplexy and other associated symptoms in some reports, but have not been studied as extensively.[29,30] SSRIs are not FDA approved for the treatment of narcolepsy. Like TCAs, they suppress REM sleep and can lead to increased cataplexy or even status cataplecticus if acutely withdrawn. Their main advantage is an improved side effect profile and lesser toxicity in comparison to TCAs. Common side effects include sexual dysfunction, headaches, gastrointestinal complaints, and insomnia with these medications. Venlafaxine may be associated with hypertension. In general, all antidepressants have the risk of precipitating a manic episode in bipolar patients, and may be associated with increased suicidality.

Sodium oxybate is the drug name for sodium salt of gamma-hydroxybutyric acid (GHB). An analogue of GABA, it binds to $GABA_B$ receptors and possibly GHB receptors in the brain.[31] When prescribed for narcolepsy, it is an FDA Schedule III substance. Sodium oxybate causes an increase in slow-wave sleep and delta EEG power, decreases daytime sleepiness, and reduces cataplexy; it can also increase the incidence of sleepwalking, probably related to its effects on slow-wave sleep. Side effects include sedation, headache, nausea, dizziness, and urinary incontinence. It can also cause respiratory depression and brady-cardia and has synergistic effects with CNS depressants and alcohol, which have led to its use as a "date rape drug." It has also been associated with abuse, dependence, and withdrawal; abrupt discontinuation can cause symptoms of tremors, tachycardia, hallucinations, delirium, rhabdomyolysis, and seizures.[32] Almost all of the patients who received sodium oxybate during clinical trials were receiving CNS stimulants. Sodium oxybate is available only through a centralized pharmacy distribution program, following patient and clinician education and proper documentation.

Since stimulants and sodium oxybate have significant adverse effects as well as potential for abuse, a physician should carefully monitor their use, including the efficacy of therapy and side effects such as cardiovascular or metabolic ab-normalities. Patients should be given the lowest dose of medication needed to reduce their symptoms, since in some cases tolerance may develop and dose increases may be needed. Patients who do not respond to stimulants or who develop increased sleepiness after previously responding to treatment should be assessed for the presence of other sleep disorders (e.g., sleep apnea, cir-cadian rhythm disorders, and periodic limb movements) or insufficient sleep. General guidelines for treatment are provided in Table 5.5, recommended guidelines for the use of stimulants are provided in Table 5.6, and information on specific medications is provided in Table 5.7. Drugs to treat cataplexy are listed in Table 5.8.

Table 5.5 Treatment of Disorders of Excessive Sleepiness

- Verify adequate hours of sleep and regular sleep schedule. Consider scheduled naps if helpful (e.g., in narcolepsy).
- Treat underlying disorders (medical, psychiatric, substance abuse) that contribute to sleepiness.
- Eliminate/minimize use of sedating medications if possible.
- Stimulant treatment for narcolepsy, idiopathic hypersomnia. Consider use in other disorders.
- Use of anticataplectic medications if needed in narcolepsy.

Table 5.6 Stimulant Medications Guidelines

- Use lowest effective dose.
- Medications should be taken on an empty stomach for better efficacy.
- Monitor effects regularly, including potential cardiovascular and metabolic side effects, no less than every 6 months for patients on chronic stimulant therapy.
- Repeated dosing during the day may be needed to maintain wakefulness, but avoid dosing late in the day to prevent insomnia at night.
- Short-acting agents may be added to longer-acting agents in some situations, such as to promote more rapid onset of effects or to improve alertness during problematic times of the day (e.g., after lunch).

Table 5.7 Stimulants

Drug	Dosage			Effects		Regulation	Side Effects
	Starting and Dose Range (mg)	Dosing†	Maximum daily dose	Half-life	Peak plasma level	FDA	
Modafinil	100–400 mg	qd or bid	600 mg	15 h	2–4 h	IV	Headache, nausea, dizziness, chest pain, arrhythmia, increased blood pressure, nervousness, insomnia, reduced efficacy of oral contraceptives. Rare: serious rash, Stevens-Johnson syndrome, angiodema
Armodafinil	50–250 mg	qd		15 h	2 h	IV	
Methylphenidate extended-release	20–60 mg	qd or bid	80 mg	2–4 h	3–7 h	II	Headache, nausea, dizziness, palpitations, tachycardia, increased blood pressure, nervousness, insomnia, irritability, mania, psychosis, dry mouth, weight loss, anorexia, rash, tics
Methylphenidate extended-release (Concerta)	18–54 mg	qd	72 mg	3–4 h	6–10 h	II	
Dextroamphetamine	5–60 mg	qd or bid		12 h	3 h	II	
Dextroamphetamine extended-release	10–60 mg	qd or bid		12 h	8 h	II	
Amphetamine/ dextroamphetamine	5–60 mg	qd or bid		d-amphetamine 10 h	3 h	II	

Amphetamine/dextroamphetamine extended-release	10–60 mg	qd		l-amphetamine 13 h	7 h	II	
Lisdexamphetamine*	30–70 mg	qd	70 mg	4 h	3.8 h (dextroamphetamine)	II	
Methamphetamine	5–40 mg	qd or bid		10 h	3–4 h	II	
Selegiline	5–40 mg	qd or bid	100 mg	8–10 h	<1 h	N/A	Warning: Combination with tyramine-containing foods, narcotics, MAO inhibitors, tricyclics, SSRIs, and stimulants can cause serious CNS toxicity. Side effects: Headache, nausea, dizziness, abdominal pain, dry mouth, insomnia.

*Lisdexamphetamine is a prodrug of dextroamphetamine.

†BID dosing should typically occur in the morning and midday.

Table 5.8 Drugs to Treat Cataplexy

Drug	Dosage			Effects		Regulation	Side Effects
	Starting and Dose Range (mg)	Dosing	Maximum daily dose	Half-life	Peak plasma level	FDA	
Sodium oxybate*	2.25–4.5 g	Bedtime, and repeat 2–4 h later	9 g	0.5–1 h	0.5–1.25 h	III	Sleep walking, confusional arousals, hallucinations, agitation, problems with bowel or bladder control, depression, nausea, tremors, blurred vision, allergic reactions
Fluoxetine	10–20 mg	qd	40 mg	4–6 days	6–8 h		GI upset, sexual dysfunction, anxiety, agitation, increased suicide risk
Venlafaxine (also extended-release)	37.5–150 mg	qd	300 mg	5 h (11 h for extended-release)	5.5 h (venlafaxine), 9 h (0–desmethyl-venlafaxine)		Anxiety, hypertension, sexual dysfunction, increased suicide risk
Protriptyline	2.5–20 mg	qd-tid	60 mg	54–92 h	8–12 h		Anticholinergic effects (blurred vision, dry mouth, urinary retention, orthostatic hypotension), flushing, tachycardia, confusion, weight gain, lowering of seizure threshold, sweating, liver toxicity
Clomipramine	75–125 mg	qd	300 mg	19–37 h	2–6 h		
Desipramine	25–200 mg	qd	200 mg	23 h	4–6 h		
Imipramine	25–200 mg	qd	300 mg	11–25 h	2–6 h		

*Also improves daytime sleepiness.

When to Refer to a Sleep Specialist

Patients with excessive sleepiness that persists despite assessment and treatment for insufficient sleep and comorbid medical and psychiatric disorders, those with suspected primary sleep disorders such as apnea or narcolepsy, or those for whom sleep testing is needed should be referred for further evaluation by a sleep specialist.

References

1. Ohayon MM. From wakefulness to excessive sleepiness: what we know and still need to know. Sleep Med Rev. 2008;12(2):129–41.

2. Ford DE, Kamerow DB. Epidemiologic study of sleep disturbance and psychiatric disorders: An opportunity for prevention? JAMA. 1989;262(11):1479–84.

3. Breslau N, Roth T, Rosenthal L, et al. Sleep disturbance and psychiatric disorders: a longitudinal epidemiological study of young adults. Biol Psychiatry. 1996;39(6):411–8.

4. Kaplan KA, Harvey AG. Hypersomnia across mood disorders: A review and synthesis. Sleep Med Rev. 2009;13(4):275–85.

5. National Institute of Neurological Disorders and Stroke. Narcolepsy Fact Sheet. 2008; http://www.ninds.nih.gov/disorders/narcolepsy/detail_narcolepsy.htm Accessed Aug 1, 2008.

6. Liu X, Uchiyama M, Kim K, et al. Sleep loss and daytime sleepiness in the general adult population of Japan. Psychiatry Res. 2000;93(1):1–11.

7. Bartlett DJ, Marshall NS, Williams A, et al. Sleep health New South Wales: chronic sleep restriction and daytime sleepiness. Intern Med J. 2008;38(1):24–31.

8. Zeman A, Britton T, Douglas N, et al. Narcolepsy and excessive daytime sleepiness. BMJ. 2004;329(7468):724–8.

9. Benca RM, Obermeyer WH, Thisted RA, et al. Sleep and psychiatric disorders: a meta-analysis. Arch Gen Psychiatry. 1992;49:651–68.

10. Nishino S. Clinical and neurobiological aspects of narcolepsy. Sleep Med. 2007;8(4):373–99.

11. Thannickal TC, Moore RY, Nienhuis R, et al. Reduced number of hypocretin neurons in human narcolepsy. Neuron. 2000;27(3):469–74.

12. American Academy of Sleep Medicine. International Classification of Sleep Disorders: Diagnostic and Coding Manual, 2nd ed. Westchester, IL: American Academy of Sleep Medicine, 2005.

13. Mignot E. Genetic and familial aspects of narcolepsy. Neurology. 1998;50(2 Suppl 1):S16–22.

14. Mignot E, Lammers GJ, Ripley B, et al. The role of cerebrospinal fluid hypocretin measurement in the diagnosis of narcolepsy and other hypersomnias. Arch Neurol. 2002;59(10):1553–62.

15. Johns MW. A new method for measuring daytime sleepiness: the Epworth Sleepiness Scale. Sleep. Dec 1991;14(6):540–5.

16. Krahn LE, Pankratz VS, Oliver L, et al. Hypocretin (orexin) levels in cerebrospinal fluid of patients with narcolepsy: relationship to cataplexy and HLA DQB1*0602 status. Sleep. 2002;25(7):733–6.

17. Littner MR, Kushida C, Wise M, et al. Practice parameters for clinical use of the multiple sleep latency test and the maintenance of wakefulness test. *Sleep.* 2005;28(1):113–21.

18. Kushida CA. Countermeasures for sleep loss and deprivation. *Curr Treat Options Neurol.* 2006;8(5):361–6.

19. Morgenthaler TI, Kapur VK, Brown T, et al. Practice parameters for the treatment of narcolepsy and other hypersomnias of central origin. *Sleep.* 2007;30(12):1705–11.

20. Darwish M, Kirby M, Hellriegel ET, et al. Armodafinil and modafinil have substantially different pharmacokinetic profiles despite having the same terminal half-lives: analysis of data from three randomized, single-dose, pharmacokinetic studies. *Clin Drug Investig.* 2009;29(9):613–23.

21. Volkow ND, Fowler JS, Logan J, et al. Effects of modafinil on dopamine and dopamine transporters in the male human brain: clinical implications. *JAMA.* 2009;301(11):1148–54.

22. Cephalon. "Prescribing Information" Sheet (PDF) for Provigil. https://www.provigil.com/hcp/default.aspx. Accessed Aug 2, 2008.

23. Morgenthaler T, Kramer M, Alessi C, et al. Practice parameters for the psychological and behavioral treatment of insomnia: an update. An American Academy of Sleep Medicine report. *Sleep.* 2006;29(11):1415–9.

24. Mignot E, Nishino S. Emerging therapies in narcolepsy-cataplexy. *Sleep.* 2005;28(6):754–63.

25. Littner M, Johnson SF, McCall WV, et al. Practice parameters for the treatment of narcolepsy: an update for 2000. *Sleep.* 2001;24(4):451–66.

26. Auger RR, Goodman SH, Silber MH, et al. Risks of high-dose stimulants in the treatment of disorders of excessive somnolence: a case-control study. *Sleep.* 2005;28(6):667–72.

27. Shire US Inc. "Prescribing Information" sheet (PDF) for Adderall XR. http://www.adderallxr.com/ Accessed Aug 1, 2008.

28. Thorpy M. Therapeutic advances in narcolepsy. *Sleep Med.* 2007;8(4):427–40.

29. Wise MS, Arand DL, Auger RR, et al. Treatment of narcolepsy and other hypersomnias of central origin. *Sleep.* 2007;30(12):1712–27.

30. Izzi F, Placidi F, Marciani MG, et al. Effective treatment of narcolepsy-cataplexy with duloxetine: a report of three cases. *Sleep Med.* 2009;10(1):153–4.

31. Carter LP, Koek W, France CP. Behavioral analyses of GHB: receptor mechanisms. *Pharmacol Ther.* 2009;121(1):100–14.

32. van Noorden MS, van Dongen LC, Zitman FG, et al. Gamma-hydroxybutyrate withdrawal syndrome: dangerous but not well-known. *Gen Hosp Psychiatry.* 2009;31(4):394–6.

33. Van Hoof E, De Becker P, Lapp C, et al. Defining the occurrence and influence of alpha-delta sleep in chronic fatigue syndrome. *Am J Med Sci.* 2007;333(2):78–84.

34. Arnulf I, Zeitzer JM, File J, et al. Kleine-Levin syndrome: a systematic review of 186 cases in the literature. *Brain.* 2005;128(Pt 12):2763–76.

Chapter 6

Circadian Rhythm Sleep Disorders

Circadian rhythm sleep disorders occur when there is a misalignment between the individual's internal circadian rhythm and the external environment. This may happen when the internal circadian rhythm fails to align properly with the external light–dark cycle, such as in delayed or advanced sleep phase disorder, irregular sleep–wake rhythm, or free-running disorder. It can also be the result of an alteration in the timing of the sleep–wake cycle relative to the internal circadian rhythm in situations such as in night-shift work or jet lag. When sleep is attempted during the circadian phase of increased alertness, the individual may develop insomnia and then complain of excessive sleepiness when trying to stay awake during the circadian phase of decreased alertness. To be considered as a disorder, the misalignment of the sleep schedule and circadian rhythm must also result in impaired functioning; simply having an unusual sleep–waking schedule is not sufficient for the diagnosis of a circadian rhythm disorder, and many individuals can become entrained to schedules that may be considered abnormal by others. For example, not all night-shift workers have a shift work disorder.

Table 6.1 defines terms used in this chapter.

Delayed Sleep Phase Disorder

Description

Individuals with delayed sleep phase disorder (DSPD) have bedtimes and waking times that are at least 2 hours later than a conventional or desired schedule. In some cases, these individuals may not be able to fall asleep reliably until as late as 5 or 6 a.m. As a result, they complain of severe sleep-onset insomnia and have extreme difficulty waking up in the morning for work, school, or other scheduled activities; during weekends or holidays they often extend their sleep period several hours later than on normal school or work days, sometimes not waking up until the middle to late afternoon. In severe cases, failure in school or loss of employment may result because of an inability to wake up in the morning.

Epidemiology

DSPD is the most common circadian rhythm sleep disorder; it has a prevalence in the general adult population estimated at 0.13% to 3.1%.[1] Symptoms of later bedtimes and more difficulty waking up in the morning are more frequent in adolescents and young adults, partly as a result of their tendency to exhibit a

Table 6.1 Definitions

Actigraphy: Measurement of rest–activity patterns with a wristwatch-like device that may be worn for several weeks at a time. Some devices also record light exposure.

Chronotherapy: Moving the internal circadian rhythm into alignment with the light–dark cycle by progressively delaying (or advancing) bedtime and waking time.

Dim light melatonin onset (DLMO): Time that melatonin secretion begins to increase as measured in serial samples of blood or saliva obtained under conditions of dim light (since bright light suppresses melatonin secretion). It is considered one of the best markers of the phase of the circadian rhythm.

Period of circadian rhythm: The period of the endogenous circadian cycle, usually slightly longer than 24 hours in humans

Phase of circadian rhythm: Refers to a particular time point within the circadian cycle, such as the core body temperature minimum or maximum, DLMO, etc.

Phase advance: A relative movement of the circadian rhythm earlier relative to the external clock time or light–dark cycle

Phase delay: A relative movement of the circadian rhythm later relative to the external clock time or light–dark cycle

phase delay in their circadian rhythm as part of normal pubertal development.[2] However, prevalence estimates of true DSPD in these younger age groups (0.2–0.48%) do not appear to be greater than in adults because the delayed sleeping schedule is not necessarily related to daytime dysfunction.[2,3] The onset of DSPD is usually during late adolescence or early adulthood, however. Males generally have a tendency for a more delayed circadian preference,[4] but it is not clear whether there are significant gender differences in the actual disorder.

Increased rates of DSPD have been reported in various patient groups, including individuals with psychiatric disorders, particularly mood disorders,[5,6] and up to 10% of individuals with sleep-onset insomnia.[7] A family history of delayed bedtimes and waking times is also greater in individuals with DSPD,[6] suggesting a possible genetic component.

Pathophysiology

There are a number of theories for DSPD, although the mechanism for the disorder has not been definitively identified.[5,8] One possibility is that affected individuals have an intrinsically longer circadian period, making it difficult for them to entrain to the 24-hour light–dark cycle. Another theory is that DSPD patients are unusually sensitive to the phase-delaying effects of light in the evening and/or insensitive or simply not exposed to the early morning, phase-advancing properties of light. They may also have a decreased homeostatic response to sleep deprivation, making it difficult for them to initiate sleep in the evening when the circadian alerting propensity is still elevated. DSPD has also been associated with polymorphisms in circadian clock and other genes.

Evaluation and Diagnosis

Diagnosis of DSPD is usually based on clinical history and documentation of delayed sleep schedule through sleep logs and/or actigraphy for a minimum of 1 week.[5,9] An actigraphy recording of a patient with DSPD is shown in Figure 6.1.

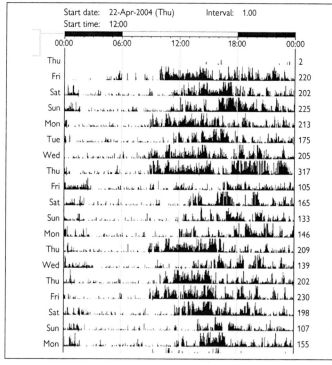

Figure 6.1 Actigraph recording from a young man with delayed sleep phase syndrome and an irregular routine. The periods of relatively low activity (sleep) vary in time placement. On most days they begin between 1 a.m. and 3 a.m. and end between 11 a.m. and noon. On some days, however, the subject had college commitments in the morning and rose at 9 a.m.

Delayed waking times may be apparent only on weekends or days without scheduled daytime obligations. Since the most prominent symptoms in patients with DSPD may be sleep-onset insomnia and/or daytime sleepiness, patients should also be screened for other sleep and medical disorders that may contribute to these symptoms. Patients should also be screened for mood or other psychiatric disorders, given the increased comorbidity of these disorders with DSPD.

Polysomnography is not routinely indicated in the evaluation except when other sleep disorders such as obstructive sleep apnea, sleep-related movement disorders, or narcolepsy are suspected. If polysomnography is performed, delayed onset of persistent sleep is usually seen, with prolonged sleep in the morning if the patient is allowed to sleep ad libitum; sleep architecture is otherwise usually normal.

Although there are currently no validated questionnaires to diagnose DSPD or other circadian rhythm disorders, patients with DSPD tend to have low scores (indicating evening phase preference) on the Morningness–Eveningness Questionnaire (MEQ)[10] (see Appendix 9).

Circadian phase markers such as the timing of melatonin secretion, measured in serial samples of saliva or plasma, have been used in clinical research studies and tend to show a phase delay.[5] However, these tests are generally not available for routine clinical use.

Treatment

Interventions for DSPD are usually aimed at shifting the circadian rhythm earlier relative to the environmental light–dark cycle, or phase-advancing the circadian rhythm. One method is to expose the patient to bright light in the morning, during the phase-advance portion of the phase-response curve (i.e., near the end of the sleep period or just upon arising in the morning, after the body temperature minimum, Fig. 6.2). Illuminance should be at least 2,500 lux with exposure for up to 2 to 3 hours.[5,11] Ideally, the patient should avoid bright light exposure from the late afternoon onward, during the time of day when light exposure would be likely to cause phase delay. This can be accomplished through use of dark goggles or sunglasses when outdoors, and avoiding exposure to bright indoor lighting or TV or computer screens in the evening. General guidelines regarding use of light therapy are listed in Table 6.2.

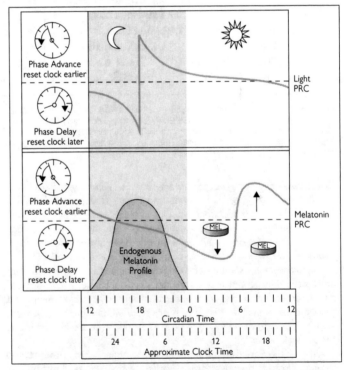

Figure 6.2 Phase-response curve for melatonin and light. Reprinted from Sack RL. The pathophysiology of jet lag. *Travel Med Infect Dis.* 2009;7(2):102–110, with permission from Elsevier.

Table 6.2 Light Therapy for Circadian Rhythm Sleep Disorders[9,42]

Light Source

- Use an apparatus capable of delivering 10,000 lux and get the largest box that is practical for the space where it will be used. This will provide the greatest therapeutic area with an illuminance level of at least 2,500 to 3,000 lux (illuminance decreases in proportion to the square of the distance from the light source).
- Fluorescent bulbs should emit white light and filter out ultraviolet irradiation.
- Light source should be positioned above eye level and angled slightly downward.

Schedule for Light Therapy

Delayed Sleep Phase Disorder
- Light exposure for at least 30 min and up to several hours upon arising in the morning.
- Avoid bright light after 4 p.m.

Advanced Sleep Phase Disorder
- Light exposure for at least 30 min and up to several hours in the evening, at or before the usual bedtime.
- Avoid bright light in the morning.

Irregular Sleep–Wake Rhythm
- Increase light exposure throughout the day (at least 1,500 lux).
- Minimize light exposure at night.

Nonentrained Type
Same as for delayed sleep phase disorder.

Jet Lag Disorder
- To prepare for eastward travel, advance bedtime by 1 hour earlier each night for 3 nights and use bright light for at least several hours upon arising in the morning.
- No studies have been performed for westward travel, but presumably evening light exposure and delayed bedtime would be effective.
- Upon arrival, increase light exposure in the morning after eastward travel (except not the first several days if more than eight time zones crossed); increase light exposure in the afternoon after westward travel.

Shift Work Disorder
- For night-shift work, intermittent periods of at least 20–30 minutes during the shift, or continuous exposure for as long as possible during the shift
- Minimize light exposure in the morning following night-shift work and in the bedroom during daytime sleep.

Adverse Effects

- Light therapy should not be used in individuals who are being treated with medications that cause photosensitivity (e.g., some antiarrhythmics, antibiotics, antidepressants, and antipsychotics) since this may cause skin reactions and/or retinal damage.
- Light therapy should not be used in individuals with macular degeneration or retinopathy.
- Side effects may include eyestrain, headache, nausea, irritability, insomnia.
- Episodes of hypomania or mania may be triggered in bipolar patients.

Sources:

Morgenthaler TI, Lee-Chiong T, Alessi C, et al. Practice parameters for the clinical evaluation and treatment of circadian rhythm sleep disorders. An American Academy of Sleep Medicine report. *Sleep.* 2007;30(11):1445–59.

Terman M, Terman J. Light therapy. In: Kryger M, Roth T, Dement W, eds. *Principles and Practice of Sleep Medicine*, 4th ed. Philadelphia, PA: Elsevier, 2005:1424–42.

Melatonin has also been shown to be effective in phase-advancing the circadian rhythm when administered in the early evening (see Fig. 6.1). The optimal dose and timing for melatonin has not been established, but phase advances have been produced with doses ranging from 0.3 to 5 mg, administered prior to sleep onset, with the maximal phase-advancing effect occurring about 6 hours before the normal onset of melatonin secretion in the evening (i.e., in the late afternoon in individuals with normal sleep patterns; melatonin secretion typically starts around 2 hours before sleep onset).[5,12,13] Of the two interventions, the phase-shifting effect of light is at least two to five times greater than for melatonin,[14] but the two may be used together. The use of melatonin for circadian rhythm disorders is outlined in Table 6.3.

Although not approved by the FDA for this indication, ramelteon, a melatonin receptor agonist, has also been shown to induce circadian phase shifts, although in doses lower than typically used for insomnia. Doses of 1 to 4 mg resulted in phase advances of 80.5 to 90.5 minutes in healthy adults.[15]

An older approach to establishing a more normal relationship between the internal circadian rhythm and the external environment is chronotherapy.[16] This technique takes advantage of the fact that patients with DSPD have a much easier time delaying than advancing their sleep schedule. The patient is instructed to delay bedtime by 2 to 3 hours every day until the desired bedtime is reached. However, unless the sleep schedule is rigidly enforced after reaching their target, patients tend to relapse and may need to repeat the

---

Table 6.3 Melatonin and Circadian Rhythm Disorders[9,26,43]

Facts about Normal Melatonin Secretion

- Melatonin is a hormone produced by the pineal gland, and its secretion is under circadian control; it acts on the suprachiasmatic nucleus (SCN) to produce circadian phase shifts (via MT2 receptors) and can also suppress SCN activity (via MT1 receptors).
- It is secreted only during the night, but its secretion is inhibited by light exposure; it is not secreted during the daytime, even in the absence of light.
- Secretion normally begins about 2 hours before usual bedtime and ceases in the morning.
- Duration of secretion is longer in the winter at more extreme latitudes due to longer night.

Melatonin as a Supplement

- Melatonin is considered a nutritional supplement and is not regulated by the FDA.
- There is a lack of standardization, so purity and reliability of dosage in various preparations may vary.
- Formulations that have a "good laboratory practice" (GLP) stamp are considered most reliable.
- Lower doses (e.g., 0.5 mg) are usually sufficient for circadian phase-shifting effects. Larger doses may be less effective for phase shifting because they can be active during both the phase-delay and phase-advance portions of the melatonin phase-response curve (see Fig. 6.1).
- Sleep-inducing effects may require higher doses of melatonin (e.g., 5 mg or more).

Table 6.3 (continued)

- Doses of 3 mg or more produce melatonin blood levels that are up to 10-fold higher than physiological levels.
- Effects of chronic melatonin use are not known, but no significant risks have been identified.
- Common side effects include headache, dizziness, drowsiness, nausea, and nightmares.
- Melatonin should not be used by women who are pregnant, planning to become pregnant, or nursing, since it may affect reproductive hormones. It may also reduce sperm count in men.
- Melatonin should not be used in individuals taking anticoagulants.

Sources:

Arendt J. Melatonin: characteristics, concerns, and prospects. *J Biol Rhythms*. 2005;20(4):291–303.

Morgenthaler TI, Lee-Chiong T, Alessi C, et al. Practice parameters for the clinical evaluation and treatment of circadian rhythm sleep disorders. An American Academy of Sleep Medicine report. *Sleep*. 2007;30(11):1445–59.

Sack RL, Auckley D, Auger RR, et al. Circadian rhythm sleep disorders: part I, basic principles, shift work and jet lag disorders. An American Academy of Sleep Medicine review. *Sleep*. 2007;30(11):1460–83.

therapy. Furthermore, the treatment may be difficult for some patients in that the schedule must be adhered to strictly, which requires that they will have the bulk of their sleep period during the normal work or school day time for a period of time. There are currently no controlled clinical trials demonstrating efficacy, but it may be a useful option for some patients, including those who fail phase-advancing treatments. Instructions for chronotherapy are listed in Table 6.4.

The choice of treatment depends on factors such as the degree of phase delay and patient preference. In general, phase-advancing techniques may be successful in patients with less extreme delays, whereas patients with typical wake-up times at noon or later may prefer chronotherapy.[17] The treatments may be combined; after achieving an appropriate sleep schedule through chronotherapy, the schedule may be reinforced with early-evening administration of melatonin and/or early-morning bright light therapy.

Additional behavioral measures include avoidance of naps, since these may serve to delay bedtime and exacerbate the problem, and regular exercise, preferably earlier in the day; exercise later in the day can contribute to phase delay. Obviously, use of stimulants that can worsen sleep-onset insomnia such as caffeine should be minimized; they should be used only in the morning.

Although stimulants and hypnotics have been used to try to regulate sleep and wakefulness in patients with DSPD, there is no evidence at present that either is efficacious or safe for this indication.

In general, DSPD can be difficult to treat and patients frequently relapse. As a result, it is important to advise patients to try to make appropriate adjustments in their life, work, or school schedules to accommodate their delayed biological clock.

Table 6.4 Chronotherapy Instructions
• Determine average bedtime and waking time from at least 1 week of sleep log data.
• Delay bedtime and waking time by 3 hours per day every day until target schedule is reached. The target schedule should be about 1–2 hours earlier than the actual desired schedule, to allow for some further delay that may occur during the stabilization period.
• Enforce a regular bedtime and waking time; staying up late for any reason can lead to a relapse.
• Consider reinforcement of new schedule with other interventions such as morning bright light, avoidance of bright light in the evening, and evening administration of melatonin.
• If relapse occurs, repeat the treatment.
• In rare cases, patients may develop free-running type disorder.

Advanced Sleep Phase Disorder

Description

Advanced sleep phase disorder (ASPD) is characterized by sleep onset and morning awakening times that are several hours earlier than normal; sleep onset usually occurs between 6 and 9 p.m. and waking times are as early as 2 to 5 a.m.[18] These patients typically complain of excessive sleepiness in the afternoon and early evening and insomnia in the early morning (early-morning awakening), with difficulty extending sleep to more "normal" wake-up times. As a result, they may become sleep-deprived due to staying up past their desired bedtime and inability to extend sleep in the morning.

Epidemiology

The prevalence of ASPD is assumed to be much lower than DSPD, but in part this could be due to the fact that ASPD may be less likely than DSPD to interfere with daytime activities such as work or school. There have been several reports of families with ASPD in which the disorder showed an autosomal dominant pattern of inheritance, and symptoms of ASPD appear to be more common in older individuals.[5,19] It is not known if there are gender-related differences in prevalence.

Pathophysiology

The mechanism(s) for ASPD are not known, but could include explanations similar to those proposed for DSPD. For example, a shortened period of the endogenous circadian rhythm could result in difficulty entraining to the 24-hour light–dark cycle. Patients with ASPD could be insensitive or not sufficiently exposed to the phase-delaying effects of light late in the day and/or hypersensitive to the phase-advancing effects in the morning.

   Studies in families with ASPD have identified mutations in circadian clock-related genes *hPer2* and *CK1δ*.[20] Defects in either of these genes can contribute to shortening the endogenous period of the clock, and it is possible that other mutations related to the regulation of circadian rhythms may be identified in familial cases.

Evaluation and Diagnosis

Diagnosis is usually based on clinical history and sleep logs and/or actigraphy for a minimum of 1 week to document early bedtimes and rise times. Patients may show evidence of sleep restriction and symptoms of sleep deprivation because daytime activities or obligations may keep them up past their desired bedtime and they are unable to extend their sleep in the morning. Patient should be assessed for other causes of daytime sleepiness or early-morning insomnia including primary sleep disorders, medical disorders, and psychiatric illnesses such as depression. Polysomnography is indicated only when other sleep disorders are suspected; if performed, it will usually show short sleep latency and early-morning awakening but generally normal sleep architecture.

Although not specifically indicated for diagnostic evaluation, circadian phase markers such as dim light melatonin onset will show a phase advance of the melatonin rhythm. The MEQ score will be high, indicating morning trait or preference.

Treatment

Treatment interventions for ASPD are similar to those used for DSPD but in the opposite direction. Light therapy is administered in the evening, with most studies using illuminance levels ranging from 2,000 to 10,000 lux and exposing patients for up to several hours, usually beginning about 8 p.m. or shortly before the habitual bedtime.[5] No controlled studies using melatonin have been performed, but data on the phase-shifting effects of melatonin suggest that early-morning administration might be useful. If administered in the early morning, patients should be started on low doses (0.1–0.3 mg) to avoid daytime sedation or other side effects.

Chronotherapy, consisting of advancing bedtime progressively until the desired schedule is reached, may also be considered, but there is only one case report describing this treatment for ASPD.[21]

Sleep hygiene recommendations include avoiding bright light or vigorous exercise early in the morning to prevent further circadian phase advance; exercise should occur in the later afternoon or even early evening.

Irregular Sleep–Wake Rhythm

Description

Patients with irregular sleep–wake rhythm (ISWR) have disorganized sleep patterns without obvious evidence of a circadian rhythm of sleep and wakefulness. Although total daily sleep time may be fairly normal, sleep is broken up into at least three major segments plus multiple naps across the 24-hour period, without a clear, consolidated period of nocturnal sleep.

Epidemiology and Pathophysiology

The prevalence is not known, but the disorder has been described in patients with dementia or retardation.[5] In these cases, it may be related to damage to the suprachiasmatic nucleus (SCN) and/or its output pathways. Factors such as retinal degeneration, decreased light exposure, and reduced activity levels during the daytime in institutionalized patients may further contribute to symptomatology.

Neurologically normal individuals may also develop ISWR, but this is usually due to extremely poor sleep hygiene. It may be more prevalent in people with relatively little daytime structure, such as individuals who live in social isolation or those with chronic medical or psychiatric disorders.

Studies have suggested a decreased amplitude of the circadian rhythm in patients with ISWR, but there is no consistent evidence of a phase advance or delay.

Evaluation and Diagnosis

Diagnosis is usually based on clinical history. In subjects who cannot maintain a reliable sleep log or diary, actigraphy may be helpful to document the sleep pattern; an example of a patient with ISWR is shown in Figure 6.3. Although

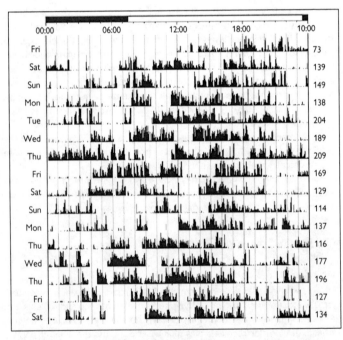

Figure 6.3 Irregular sleep–wake rhythm. Actigraph showing irregular routine in an alcoholic person who had been abstinent for 2 weeks. There are no consistent sleeping and waking times, with naps and short sleeps interspersed with varying levels of waking activity.

polysomnography is not routinely indicated, it is useful to document the fragmented sleep pattern as well as determine whether other sleep disorders that may contribute to sleep fragmentation are present; individuals with neurodegenerative diseases are at increased risk for disorders such as apnea and sleep-related movement disorders, for example. Medication effects can also contribute to sleep fragmentation and daytime sleepiness, particularly in patients whose polypharmacy may include sedating drugs as well as medications with stimulant effects. In all cases, the patient's sleep hygiene, daily routine/activities, and light exposure should be assessed.

Treatment

Interventions for ISWR are aimed at increasing the amplitude of the circadian rhythm.[5] These include increasing bright light exposure during the daytime, administering melatonin at bedtime, and increasing daytime activity; in general, there are limited data related to these modalities but some improvements have been reported.

A variety of psychotropic medications have been used historically to try to improve nocturnal sleep in demented patients, but there are no data supporting their use in this setting. Furthermore, sedative-hypnotics, antipsychotics, sedating antidepressants, and antihistamines all have significant risks associated with their use, particularly in an elderly and demented population. Similarly, there are no data regarding the efficacy and safety of stimulants to promote daytime alertness in patients with dementia.

Free-Running Disorder

Description

The non-entrained type or free-running type of circadian rhythm disorder (free-running disorder [FRD]; also called non-24-hour sleep–wake syndrome) occurs when an individual's circadian rhythm fails to entrain to the 24-hour day. In all reported cases, the endogenous circadian rhythm was always greater than 24 hours, resulting in a gradual and continual phase delay relative to the environment. Over time, the individual's internal clock will be at different phase relationships with the external environment, resulting in periods where the pattern is similar to ASPD (falling asleep and waking up too early) or DSPD (falling asleep and waking up too late), as well as times when the sleep–wake schedule appears to be entrained properly.

Epidemiology and Pathophysiology

FRD has been described in two groups of individuals: the totally blind and individuals with normal sight. Over half of those who are totally blind (i.e., no visual light perception) may have FRD due to failure to entrain their circadian rhythms to the 24-hour light–dark cycle.[22] However, most "legally blind" individuals have light perception and are usually able to entrain normally to the light–dark cycle.

In the normally sighted, the incidence of FRD is not known. However, it typically begins in adolescence or young adulthood and may represent an exaggerated form of DSPD, in which the individual continues to delay the phase of the sleep–wake cycle relative to the environment;[23] this may be due to a long intrinsic period of the endogenous circadian rhythm, similar to DSPD.[24] In sighted individuals, the disorder is more common in males and those with psychiatric disorders.

Evaluation and Diagnosis

Clinical history and documentation of sleep–wake patterns through sleep logs or actigraphy are usually sufficient, although sleep patterns must be documented for prolonged periods of time, usually several weeks to months, to detect the free-running pattern. An example of FRD is shown in Figure 6.4. Polysomnography is not routinely performed and is indicated only to exclude other sleep disorders; if performed, it will show normal sleep architecture during the patient's usual sleep period. Sighted individuals with the disorder

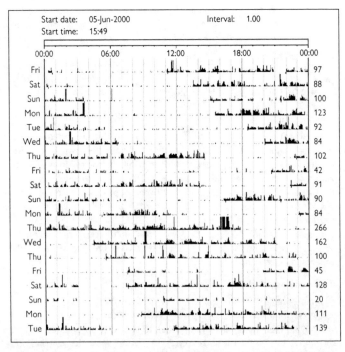

Figure 6.4 Free-running disorder. Actigraph recording of a schizophrenic patient whose sleep–wake routine was "free-running." This is a double-plot display. Note how the inactive (sleep) period runs from 12:30 to 11 a.m. at the top and gets later each day. General levels of activity during the wake period are low.

should be screened for psychiatric disorders if not already diagnosed, given the increased comorbidity, particularly with mood disorders.

Although not available for routine clinical use at present, serial determinations of circadian phase over several weeks using dim light melatonin onset will demonstrate the progressive delay in the circadian rhythm over time.

Treatment

In blind individuals, melatonin in doses ranging from 0.5 to 10 mg administered at 9 p.m. has been shown to be effective in producing stable entrainment.[5] Low-dose melatonin (0.5 mg) appears to be more effective than higher doses, particularly when melatonin treatment is initiated near the preferred bedtime (e.g., at 9 p.m.).[22]

In sighted individuals, melatonin administration also appears be effective in the few cases where it has been tried. Light therapy can also be used to entrain the circadian rhythm in these patients, and morning bright light exposure has been successful in a series of case reports.[5]

In addition to providing entraining stimuli, patients should be counseled regarding appropriate sleep hygiene, including maintaining a regular bedtime and waking time, avoiding naps, increasing physical activity during the daytime, and, for sighted individuals, increasing light exposure during the day and avoiding bright light at night. Stimulant and hypnotic medications have not been studied in these patients and are not indicated for treatment.

Jet Lag Disorder

Description

Jet lag is experienced in some degree by most individuals who travel across several time zones. It is a temporary condition that results from the mismatch between the internal circadian rhythm and the new time zone and usually resolves after several days in the new environment. Symptoms include daytime sleepiness and difficulty initiating or maintaining sleep during the night. With eastward travel, difficulty falling asleep and difficulty awakening in the morning are typically experienced, as the scheduled sleep and waking times in the new environment are several hours earlier than in the home setting. Conversely, in westward travel, individuals may have difficulty staying awake until the new, later bedtime and often have trouble maintaining sleep later in the night. In addition, individuals may complain of problems with daytime function, fatigue or malaise, decreased alertness and concentration, mood changes, and gastrointestinal upset.

For individuals who travel across time zones infrequently, such as for vacations, jet lag is usually self-limited. However, for long-haul airline crews or business travelers, frequent time zone shifts can lead to a chronic state of desynchronization of circadian rhythms, with the development of chronic symptoms of jet lag due to the failure to remain in a single time zone long enough for re-entrainment of the circadian rhythm to occur. In these cases, there may also be possible long-term health risks similar to those reported for chronic shift work (see below).

Epidemiology and Pathophysiology

Jet lag occurs because the internal circadian rhythm is no longer properly aligned with the external light–dark cycle,[25] and the severity of jet lag usually increases with the number of time zones traversed.[26] For most individuals, eastbound travel requires a longer period of adjustment than westbound travel because of the natural tendency of the circadian rhythm to phase delay. Although the sleep–wake schedule may adjust to the new time zone schedule within a few days, it may take other circadian rhythm outputs such as core body temperature and hormonal rhythms longer to resynchronize.[27]

A number of other factors may worsen jet leg, including sleep deprivation prior to travel and excessive use of caffeine or alcohol.[28] Time of arrival may also play a role, in that light exposure in the destination could exert a phase-shifting effect on the circadian clock in the wrong direction; for example, with eastward travel, arrival in the early morning may expose the individual to a phase-delaying pulse of light, whereas the needed circadian accommodation is a phase advance. Younger individuals seem to experience more severe jet lag than older adults. It is not clear if there are significant gender differences. Finally, factors such as simply spending significant time in an aircraft at high altitude may contribute to some of the associated symptoms (e.g., cognitive and psycho-motor dysfunction) through the effects of hypoxia and sleep deprivation.

Evaluation and Diagnosis

For the occasional traveler, jet lag is managed prospectively by advising patients on countermeasures to minimize the effects of travel across time zones (see next section). Chronic jet lag may be diagnosed by history in patients who travel frequently across at least two time zones. Documenting the sleep history with a sleep log or actigraphy is often helpful, and polysomnography is indicated when other sleep disorders may be present that could contribute to symp-tomatology. Patients should also be screened for other medical and psychiatric disorders that may account for their symptoms.

Treatment

Treatment of jet lag is aimed at countermeasures to minimize symptoms.[9] For brief periods of travel, it is usually not practical to attempt to entrain to the new time zone, whereas interventions to hasten entrainment may be useful for longer trips.

For trips that last only a few days, trying to stay on a sleep schedule close to the one at home may allow the traveler to obtain better-quality sleep and a greater amount of sleep.[26] Alternatively, shifting the home schedule by a few hours for several days prior to travel to more closely approximate the destina-tion schedule and then adhering to that schedule may minimize the effects of jet lag; this approach may be helpful for eastward travel, where a phase advance of the sleep schedule is required.

For longer periods of travel, circadian phase-shifting interventions that would lead to more rapid entrainment to the new time zone have been sug-gested as potentially helpful, and there are a few studies to support such interventions. More data are available regarding the efficacy of melatonin to minimize the effects of jet lag.[26,28] To facilitate entrainment to the new time zone, melatonin ranging from 0.5 to 10 mg is generally administered at the destination bedtime starting up to 3 days prior to travel, or beginning on the first night after arrival at the destination. Most studies using this dosing schedule have reported decreased symptoms of jet lag and sleep disruption. Immediate-release preparations of melatonin appeared to be more effective than delayed-release formulations, and low doses have better phase-shifting properties and reduced side effects than higher doses.

Timed light exposure is also effective in shifting circadian rhythms, and recovery from jet lag normally requires exposure to the new light–dark cycle. Bright light therapy has not been used for jet lag on a widespread basis, however, probably due to the difficulties most individuals would have strictly controlling their light exposure. Bright light combined with shifting the sleep schedule prior to travel may hasten accommodation to the destination schedule. For eastward travel, bright light exposure should occur in the early morning combined with gradually advancing bedtime and waking time for several days prior to travel. For westward travel, the opposite should occur (i.e., bright late in the evening combined with delayed bedtime and waking time). If the new time zone requires a particularly large phase advance for accommodation, it may be easier to delay the circadian clock; for example, instead of trying to advance the clock by 9 hours, it may be easier to delay by 15 hours.

Use of hypnotics or stimulants might be considered in selected cases,[26] although it is important to be aware that the Federal Aviation Administration forbids use of these substances by active-duty airline personnel. Hypnotics are often used acutely to treat the insomnia associated with jet lag and are indicated as for any transient insomnia (see Chapter 3, section on pharmacotherapy, and Table 3.10). Hypnotics should be used with extreme caution if at all on long-distance flights because they have been associated with confusion or amnestic responses and could increase the risk for deep vein thrombosis due to inactivity.

The primary stimulant used to counteract jet lag is caffeine, and although it may lead to improved alertness and daytime function, it can also exacerbate insomnia during periods of jet lag. If used to diminish daytime sleepiness, it should not be used later in the day, to minimize disruption of sleep. Use of prescription stimulants is not indicated for jet lag. Caffeine has a half-life of about 5 hours, but this can be increased with use of oral contraceptives; the half-life is dramatically increased in patients taking fluvoxamine. In higher doses, caffeine may also produce anxiety, irritability, restlessness, agitation, gastrointestinal upset, diuresis, tachycardia, palpitations, arrhythmia, and muscle twitching. Withdrawal symptoms, consisting of increased fatigue and drowsiness, headache, irritability, depression, and aches and pains may last up to several days.

General recommendations for treating jet lag are listed in Table 6.5.

Table 6.5 Countermeasures to Reduce Jet Lag

Short-Duration Travel (2 days or less at destination)
- Avoid sleep deprivation prior to departure.
- Avoid use of alcohol or caffeine in flight.
- Consider keeping home-based sleep schedule, or a sleep schedule that largely overlaps with home-based schedule.
- Consider use of hypnotic for insomnia.

Longer-Duration Travel
Prior to travel
- Avoid sleep deprivation.
- For eastward travel, shift waking time and bedtime earlier by 1 hour per day for 3 days prior to departure; use bright light early in the morning to advance the circadian rhythm and avoid light exposure late in the day. Maximal phase advance occurs with light treatment begun approximately 1 hour before or at typical waking time.[44]
- For westward travel, shift bedtime and waking time later for several days prior to travel; use bright light in the evening or during the first part of the night to delay the circadian rhythm and avoid light exposure in the morning. Maximal phase delay occurs with light exposure approximately 3–4 hours after typical bedtime.[44]
- Consider use of low-dose melatonin (0.5–5 mg) at the anticipated bedtime in the destination.

In flight
- Avoid use of alcohol and caffeine.
- Try to sleep.

Upon arrival
- Adapt to the schedule in the new time zone by remaining awake during the daytime and following the new mealtimes.
- For eastward travel, increase light exposure in the morning. For travel across more than three or four time zones, avoid light exposure for the first few hours of the morning for the first 2 days and increase light exposure during the later morning/midday. After 2 days, increase early-morning light exposure.
- For westward travel, increase light exposure in the late afternoon/evening and minimize light exposure in the morning. For travel across more than eight time zones, avoid light in the few hours before sunset for 2 days.
- Consider use of low-dose melatonin (0.5–5 mg) at bedtime.
- For insomnia, consider short-term use of a hypnotic.
- Caffeine may be used to counteract daytime sleepiness but should be avoided within 8 hours of bedtime.

Shift Work Disorder

Description

Shift work sleep disorder (SWD) can occur when individuals are required to work during their normal sleep hours and sleep during normal waking hours. As a result, shift workers may report difficulty staying awake and alert on the job and difficulty sleeping during the day. Daytime sleep is often shortened, not only due to the inability to sleep resulting from the circadian misalignment, but also because of other factors such as daytime demands or interruptions (e.g., family duties, social interactions, appointments, telephone calls). For example, a recent study in nurses found that sleep amount was decreased by about 40% during periods of night shift work compared to working during the day.[29]

Other symptoms of SWD include impaired performance, increased risk of accidents, irritability, and mood disturbance. Chronic shift workers also appear to be at increased risk for various health problems, including gastrointestinal complaints, ulcers, cardiovascular disease, depression, breast cancer, metabolic syndrome, and alcohol and drug use/abuse.[30-32]

Epidemiology and Pathophysiology

Up to 20% of U.S. workers are involved in some kind of shift work,[9] including individuals who work during the night or start work unusually early in the morning. In addition to factory workers, shift workers include individuals in critical industries and services such as health care, police and fire departments, transportation, energy, and the military. It is estimated that 26% of rotating shift workers and 32% of night-shift workers may have at least some symptoms of SWD, although the true prevalence of SWD in shift workers is probably about 10%.[30]

Older individuals appear to be less tolerant of shift work, and there are some suggestions that women may be at greater risk for SWD. Other sleep disorders or sleep deprivation may exacerbate SWD as well. The shift work schedule is also a factor, in that rotating shift work is more problematic when the shifts advance rather than delay;[33] this is because the natural tendency for most individuals is to delay their circadian rhythm (e.g., go to bed and wake up later). Long-duration shifts are also problematic in that they compound the problems of circadian misalignment with the added component of sleep deprivation, thereby increasing risks for mistakes and accidents. These risks are particularly problematic in professions where safety is critical, such as health care, transportation, and the military.[34]

Without interventions, most shift workers end up being exposed to sunlight, either going to and from work or on days off, and for many of them, their circadian rhythms remain relatively entrained to the normal light–dark cycle and do not shift to become fully synchronized with the desired sleep–wake pattern. Thus SWD is usually a chronic condition (unlike jet lag, in which the circadian rhythm eventually shifts to the new schedule).

Evaluation and Diagnosis

The diagnosis of SWD is based on clinical history and evaluation in an individual who has a history of performing shift work. Some data suggest that individuals who are extreme morning types as measured on the MEQ may have a more difficult time adjusting to shift work, although the MEQ is not diagnostically specific for this purpose. Sleep logs or actigraphy may be helpful for documenting sleep patterns and determining appropriate treatment recommendations. Polysomnography is not indicated for routine evaluation of SWD, but it may be performed if other primary sleep disorders such as sleep apnea are suspected. If a sleep study is required in a regular night-shift worker, performance of the study during the daytime should be considered. For patients with SWD, a sleep study performed during their usual scheduled sleep period may show prolonged latency to sleep onset, fragmented sleep, and/or decreased duration of total sleep.

Treatment

The shift work schedule may provide an opportunity for intervention in some cases. In general, workers assigned to rotating shifts adapt better to shifts that progressively delay than advance. Longer shifts that contribute to sleep deprivation are associated with worse outcomes in terms of performance, health, and safety, particularly in critical occupations.[34,35] For night-shift workers who become progressively more sleep-deprived by working many nights in a row, breaking up consecutive work days with days off may be beneficial. In many cases, these are not variables that can be easily altered, but they should be assessed.

Treatment strategies for SWD are aimed at improving the alignment of the circadian rhythm with the work/sleep schedule as well as interventions to improve waking function and sleep.[9,26] Several strategies have been demonstrated to improve circadian alignment in night-shift workers, such that some individuals can become completely re-entrained to the night-shift schedule.[36] Increasing light exposure during the night through use of intermittent light pulses (2,350–12,000 lux) for at least half of the work shift has been shown to improve waking performance and shift circadian rhythms.[9,36] Additional interventions that may help include minimizing light exposure on the way home and during the sleep period through use of dark goggles and blackout window shades, and use of melatonin prior to daytime sleep. Complete re-entrainment of the circadian rhythm, however, is not necessary for improving daytime sleep and nighttime performance by these interventions, nor is the ability to shift the circadian rhythm to the new schedule indicative of shift work tolerance.

Another strategy that can improve alertness and performance in night-shift workers is to take a nap before the scheduled shift, or during the shift if this is possible. Sleep deprivation should be avoided in shift workers, since this will exacerbate sleepiness, particularly during the low point of the circadian alerting signal, usually in the early morning.

Melatonin administration during the daytime may be useful to help promote sleep as well as shift circadian rhythms. Hypnotics may also be useful for insomnia associated with daytime sleep (see Table 3.10). In general, it is preferable to start with a shorter-acting agent and switch to longer-acting medications only if sleep maintenance continues to be a problem and if there are not hangover effects that may worsen sleepiness or performance on the job.

To improve alertness during the night shift, stimulant medication may be needed in some cases of SWD. Caffeine, modafinil, and armodafinil are preferred choices, as there are at least some data supporting their use and their safety profile is preferable to amphetamines and other stimulants. Both modafinil and armodafinil have FDA indications for use in SWD and have been demonstrated to improve alertness and performance and decrease sleepiness;[37,38] the magnitude of improvement in objective sleepiness as measured by the Multiple Sleep Latency Test was greater in the armodafinil study, but there has not been a direct comparison of the two drugs for this purpose. Caffeine is commonly used by shift workers, and studies suggest that doses of about 4 mg/kg body weight (or 300–400 mg) at the beginning of the night shift improve alertness and performance;[39] the combination of napping prior to the night shift and caffeine appeared to be better than napping or caffeine alone. Stimulants other than caffeine and armodafinil/modafinil have not been studied systematically in SWD, and there are increased risks associated with their use. If used, stimulants should be taken at the beginning of the shift so as to minimize interference with sleep during the following day. One important caveat is that stimulants are not a substitute for sleep and should not be used to compensate for insufficient sleep.

An often-overlooked factor in SWD is the sleep schedule on work days versus days off. Night-shift workers not infrequently schedule their sleep time on days off during the night, often for social reasons such as to accommodate to their family's schedule. In many cases, their sleep schedule on days off may be shifted by as much as 12 hours from the time they sleep on work days; for some individuals this might worsen the circadian dysregulation and exacerbate sleep disturbance, particularly if they do not have more than a day or two off at a time. Although there are not specific studies addressing the optimal scheduling of sleep in shift workers, in some cases it may be preferable to have a sleep schedule on days off that overlaps at least somewhat with the typical sleep period on work days.

In some cases, the most appropriate treatment for SWD may be to have the patient adopt a regular shift during the daytime. Individuals who have severe difficulty adjusting to night-shift work or who have other medical, psychiatric, or sleep disorders that are exacerbated by shift work may need to be medically excused from night or rotating work schedules. For example, patients with significant sleep apnea may already have excessive sleepiness that makes them less tolerant of night-shift work, and the sleep deprivation associated with shift work may exacerbate their apnea.[40] Patients with bipolar disorder should probably avoid shift work as well, since the disorder is associated with abnormalities in circadian rhythms and sleep deprivation can trigger episodes of mania; stabilizing sleep patterns and social rhythms is a key component of treatment.[41] Countermeasures for shift work are described in Table 6.6.

When to Refer to a Sleep Specialist

Many cases of circadian rhythm disorders may be diagnosed and treated by primary care or mental health providers. Patients with more severe symptomatology, patients who do not respond to treatment, or patients suspected of having another sleep disorder should be referred to a sleep specialist for further evaluation.

Diagnostic criteria for circadian rhythm sleep disorders are described in Table 6.7. Diagrams of typical sleep patterns associated with the major categories of disorders are shown in Figure 6.2. Diagnostic and therapeutic approaches are listed in Table 6.8.

Table 6.6 Strategies for Shift Workers

Sleep–Wake Scheduling Interventions

- Schedule adequate hours in bed for sleep every day.
- Use days off to catch up on sleep.
- Consider decreasing number of consecutive night shifts.
- On days off, try to have sleep schedule overlap at least partially with sleep period on work days to minimize circadian dysregulation.
- For rotating shift work, have shifts rotate clockwise or in a phase-delay direction.
- Try to nap prior to a night shift, or early in the shift if possible.

Circadian Phase-Shifting Interventions

- Use bright light in the workplace if possible. This may include intermittent or continuous exposure to at least 2,000 lux.
- Use goggles or sunglasses to minimize light exposure in the morning, following night-shift work. Bedroom for daytime sleep should be dark.
- Administer melatonin prior to daytime sleep.

Pharmacotherapy

- For alertness during night shifts, consider caffeine (up to 4 mg/kg), modafinil (200–400 mg), or armodafinil (150 mg) administered 1 hour before the beginning of the shift (see Table 5.7 for more information).
- For insomnia, consider melatonin (for daytime sleep) or a hypnotic.

Table 6.7 Diagnostic Criteria for Circadian Rhythm Disorders

General Criteria for All Disorders

- Persistent or recurrent sleep disturbance due to alteration of the circadian timekeeping system or misalignment between the endogenous circadian rhythm and exogenous factors that affect timing or duration of sleep
- Disorder causes insomnia, excessive sleepiness, or both.
- Associated with impairment of social, occupational, or other functioning

Circadian Rhythm Sleep Disorder, Delayed Sleep Phase Type (Delayed Sleep Phase Disorder)

- Delay in the occurrence of the sleep period in relation to the desired or normal bedtime and wake-up time, associated with inability to fall asleep (sleep-onset insomnia) and difficulty waking up in the morning
- When allowed to choose their own schedule, patients will have a stable but phase-delayed pattern of sleep, with normal sleep quality and duration.
- Sleep log or actigraphy for at least 7 days demonstrates a stable delay in the timing of the sleep period; this may be confirmed by measurement of the circadian rhythm through measurement of core body temperature minimum or melatonin onset.

Table 6.7 (Continued)

Circadian Rhythm Sleep Disorder, Advanced Sleep Phase Type (Advanced Sleep Phase Disorder)

• Advance in the occurrence of the sleep period in relation to the desired or normal bedtime and wake-up time, associated with inability to stay awake until desired bedtime and difficulty remaining asleep (early-morning awakening)

• When allowed to choose their own schedule, patients will have a stable but phase-advanced pattern of sleep, with normal sleep quality and duration.

• Sleep log or actigraphy for at least 7 days demonstrates a stable advance in the timing of the sleep period; this may be confirmed by measurement of the circadian rhythm through measurement of core body temperature minimum or melatonin onset.

Circadian Rhythm Sleep Disorder, Irregular Sleep–Wake Type (Irregular Sleep–Wake Rhythm)

• Complaint of chronic insomnia, excessive sleepiness, or both

• Sleep log or actigraphy for at least 7 days demonstrates multiple (at least 3) irregular sleep bouts during each 24-hour period.

• Total daily sleep time is normal for age.

Circadian Rhythm Sleep Disorder, Free-Running Type (Non-entrained Type)

• Complaints of insomnia and hypersomnia related to mismatch between the endogenous circadian rhythm and external light–dark cycle, which may change over time as the relation between the internal rhythm and light–dark cycle changes.

• Sleep log or actigraphy for at least 7 days (preferably several weeks) demonstrates progressive delay of the sleep and wake times, with a period of >24 hours.

Circadian Rhythm Sleep Disorder, Jet Lag Type (Jet Lag Disorder)

• Insomnia or excessive sleepiness related to jet travel across at least two time zones

• Associated impairment of daytime function, malaise, or gastrointestinal disturbance for several days after travel

Circadian Rhythm Sleep Disorder, Shift Work Type (Shift Work Disorder)

• Insomnia or excessive sleepiness lasting at least 1 month and related to a work schedule that overlaps the normal sleep schedule

• Sleep log or actigraphy for at least 7 days shows disturbed circadian rhythm and sleep-time misalignment.

Circadian Rhythm Sleep Disorder due to Medical Condition

• A circadian rhythm sleep disorder (see general criteria above) that is predominantly accounted for by an underlying medical or neurological disorder (e.g., dementia)

• Sleep log or actigraphy for at least 7 days shows disturbed or low-amplitude circadian rhythmicity.

Other Circadian Rhythm Sleep Disorder (Circadian Rhythm Disorder, NOS)

• A circadian rhythm sleep disorder that is not caused by a drug or substance and does not meet criteria for another circadian rhythm disorder

Other Circadian Rhythm Sleep Disorder Due to Drug or Substance

• A circadian rhythm disorder that is due to a drug or substance

Adapted with permission from the American Academy of Sleep Medicine. *International Classification of Sleep Disorders: Diagnostic and Coding Manual*, 2nd ed. Darien, IL: American Academy of Sleep Medicine, 2005.

Table 6.8 AASM Practice Parameters for Assessment and Treatment of Circadian Rhythm Sleep Disorders

	Delayed Sleep Phase Disorder	Advanced Sleep Phase Disorder	Irregular Sleep–Wake Rhythm	Circadian Rhythm Sleep Disorder, Free-Running Type (Non-entrained Type)	Jet Lag Disorder	Shift Work Disorder
Evaluation Tools						
Polysomnography	NRI (Standard)	NRI (Standard)	NRI (Standard)	NRI (Standard)	NRI (Standard)	NRI (Standard)
Morningness–Eveningness Questionnaire (MEQ)	IE (Option)	IE (Option)	IE (Option)	IE (Option)	IE (Option)	IE (Option)
Circadian phase markers	IE (Option)	IE (Option)	IE (Option)	Indicated (Option)	IE (Option)	IE (Option)
Actigraphy for diagnosis	Indicated (Guideline)	Indicated (Guideline)	Indicated (Option)	Indicated (Option)	NRI (Option)	Indicated (Guideline)
Actigraphy for response to therapy	Indicated (Guideline)	Indicated (Guideline)	Indicated (Guideline)	Indicated (Guideline)	Indicated (Guideline)	Indicated (Guideline)
Sleep log or diary	Indicated (Guideline)	Indicated (Guideline)	Indicated (Guideline)	Indicated (Guideline)	Indicated (Guideline)	Indicated (Guideline)
Therapy						
Planned sleep schedules	Indicated (Option)	Indicated (Option)	Indicated (Option / Guideline)[1]	Indicated (Option)	Indicated (Option)	Indicated (Standard)
Timed light exposure	Indicated (Guideline)	Indicated (Option)	Indicated (Option)	Indicated (Option)	Indicated (Option)	Indicated (Guideline)
Timed melatonin administration	Indicated (Guideline)	Indicated (Option)	Indicated for (Option)[2]	Indicated (Option) / Indicated (Guideline)	Indicated (Standard)	Indicated (Guideline)

Hypnotics	NR (Option)	-	-	Indicated (Option)	Indicated (Guideline)
Stimulants	-	-	-	Indicated (Option)	Indicated (Guideline)[3] (Option)[4]
Alerting agents	-	-	-		Indicated (Guideline)[5]

NRI = Not routinely indicated; IE = Insufficient evidence to recommend; NR = Not recommended; - = No recommendation is indicated.

[1] Mixed modality behavioral therapy indicated for elderly-demented/nursing home patients including daytime bright light and physical activity, and other modalities such as sleep scheduling, structured bedtime routine, and decreased noise and light at night.

[2] Timed melatonin administration indicated for those with mental retardation, but not for elderly-demented/nursing home patients.

[3] Modafinil

[4] Caffeine

[5] Modafinil and armodafinil

Reproduced with permission: Morgenthaler TI, Lee-Chiong T, Alessi C, et al. Practice parameters for the clinical evaluation and treatment of circadian rhythm sleep disorders. Sleep 2007;30(11):1445–1459. Copyright 2007 by American Academy of Sleep Medicine.

References

1. Wyatt JK. Delayed sleep phase syndrome: pathophysiology and treatment options. *Sleep.* 2004;27(6):1195–203.

2. Crowley SJ, Acebo C, Carskadon MA. Sleep, circadian rhythms, and delayed phase in adolescence. *Sleep Med.* 2007;8(6):602–12.

3. Hazama GI, Inoue Y, Kojima K, et al. The prevalence of probable delayed-sleep-phase syndrome in students from junior high school to university in Tottori, Japan. *Tohoku J Exp Med.* 2008;216(1):95–8.

4. Roenneberg T, Kuehnle T, Pramstaller PP, et al. A marker for the end of adolescence. *Curr Biol.* 2004;14(24):R1038–9.

5. Sack RL, Auckley D, Auger RR, et al. Circadian rhythm sleep disorders: part II, advanced sleep phase disorder, delayed sleep phase disorder, free-running disorder, and irregular sleep-wake rhythm. An American Academy of Sleep Medicine review. *Sleep.* 2007;30(11):1484–501.

6. Kripke DF, Rex KM, Ancoli-Israel S, et al. Delayed sleep phase cases and controls. *J Circadian Rhythms.* 2008;6:6.

7. Weitzman ED, Czeisler CA, Coleman RM, et al. Delayed sleep phase syndrome. A chronobiological disorder with sleep-onset insomnia. *Arch Gen Psychiatry.* 1981;38(7):737–46.

8. Reid KJ, Zee PC. Circadian rhythm disorders. *Semin Neurol.* 2009;29(4):393–405.

9. Morgenthaler TI, Lee-Chiong T, Alessi C, et al. Practice parameters for the clinical evaluation and treatment of circadian rhythm sleep disorders. An American Academy of Sleep Medicine report. *Sleep.* 2007;30(11):1445–59.

10. Horne JA, Ostberg O. A self-assessment questionnaire to determine morningness-eveningness in human circadian rhythms. *Int J Chronobiol.* 1976;4(2):97–110.

11. Chesson AL, Jr., Littner M, Davila D, et al. Practice parameters for the use of light therapy in the treatment of sleep disorders. Standards of Practice Committee, American Academy of Sleep Medicine. *Sleep.* 1999;22(5):641–60.

12. Burgess HJ, Revell VL, Eastman CI. A three pulse phase response curve to three milligrams of melatonin in humans. *J Physiol.* 2008;586(2):639–47.

13. Mundey K, Benloucif S, Harsanyi K, et al. Phase-dependent treatment of delayed sleep phase syndrome with melatonin. *Sleep.* 2005;28(10):1271–8.

14. Revell VL, Eastman CI. How to trick Mother Nature into letting you fly around or stay up all night. *J Biol Rhythms.* 2005;20(4):353–65.

15. Richardson GS, Zee PC, Wang-Weigand S, et al. Circadian phase-shifting effects of repeated ramelteon administration in healthy adults. *J Clin Sleep Med.* 2008;4(5):456–61.

16. Czeisler CA, Richardson GS, Coleman RM, et al. Chronotherapy: resetting the circadian clocks of patients with delayed sleep phase insomnia. *Sleep.* 1981;4(1):1–21.

17. Lack LC, Wright HR. Clinical management of delayed sleep phase disorder. *Behav Sleep Med.* 2007;5(1):57–76.

18. American Academy of Sleep Medicine. *International Classification of Sleep Disorders: Diagnostic and Coding Manual,* 2nd ed. Westchester, IL: American Academy of Sleep Medicine, 2005.

19. Barion A, Zee PC. A clinical approach to circadian rhythm sleep disorders. *Sleep Med.* 2007;8(6):566–77.

20. Tafti M, Dauvilliers Y, Overeem S. Narcolepsy and familial advanced sleep-phase syndrome: molecular genetics of sleep disorders. *Curr Opin Genet Dev.* 2007;17(3):222–7.

21. Moldofsky H, Musisi S, Phillipson EA. Treatment of a case of advanced sleep phase syndrome by phase advance chronotherapy. *Sleep.* 1986;9(1):61–5.

22. Lockley SW, Arendt J, Skene DJ. Visual impairment and circadian rhythm disorders. *Dialogues Clin Neurosci.* 2007;9(3):301–14.

23. Uchiyama M, Okawa M, Shibui K, et al. Altered phase relation between sleep timing and core body temperature rhythm in delayed sleep phase syndrome and non-24-hour sleep-wake syndrome in humans. *Neurosci Lett.* 2000;294(2):101–4.

24. Hayakawa T, Uchiyama M, Kamei Y, et al. Clinical analyses of sighted patients with non-24-hour sleep-wake syndrome: a study of 57 consecutively diagnosed cases. *Sleep.* 2005;28(8):945–52.

25. Sack RL. The pathophysiology of jet lag. *Travel Med Infect Dis.* 2009;7(2):102–10.

26. Sack RL, Auckley D, Auger RR, et al. Circadian rhythm sleep disorders: part I, basic principles, shift work and jet lag disorders. An American Academy of Sleep Medicine review. *Sleep.* 2007;30(11):1460–83.

27. Coste O, Lagarde D. Clinical management of jet lag: what can be proposed when performance is critical? *Travel Med Infect Dis.* 2009;7(2):82–87.

28. Auger RR, Morgenthaler TI. Jet lag and other sleep disorders relevant to the traveler. *Travel Med Infect Dis.* 2009;7(2):60–8.

29. Grundy A, Sanchez M, Richardson H, et al. Light intensity exposure, sleep duration, physical activity, and biomarkers of melatonin among rotating shift nurses. *Chronobiol Int.* 2009;26(7):1443–61.

30. Drake CL, Roehrs T, Richardson G, et al. Shift work sleep disorder: prevalence and consequences beyond that of symptomatic day workers. *Sleep.* 2004;27(8):1453–62.

31. Kolstad HA. Nightshift work and risk of breast cancer and other cancers—a critical review of the epidemiologic evidence. *Scand J Work Environ Health.* 2008;34(1):5–22.

32. Karlsson B, Knutsson A, Lindahl B. Is there an association between shift work and having a metabolic syndrome? Results from a population based study of 27,485 people. *Occup Environ Med.* 2001;58(11):747–52.

33. Driscoll TR, Grunstein RR, Rogers NL. A systematic review of the neurobehavioural and physiological effects of shiftwork systems. *Sleep Med Rev.* 2007;11(3):179–94.

34. Barger LK, Lockley SW, Rajaratnam SM, et al. Neurobehavioral, health, and safety consequences associated with shift work in safety-sensitive professions. *Curr Neurol Neurosci Rep.* 2009;9(2):155–64.

35. Goel N, Rao H, Durmer JS, et al. Neurocognitive consequences of sleep deprivation. *Semin Neurol.* 2009;29(4):320–39.

36. Crowley SJ, Lee C, Tseng CY, et al. Combinations of bright light, scheduled dark, sunglasses, and melatonin to facilitate circadian entrainment to night shift work. *J Biol Rhythms.* 2003;18(6):513–23.

37. Czeisler CA, Walsh JK, Roth T, et al. Modafinil for excessive sleepiness associated with shift-work sleep disorder. *N Engl J Med.* 2005;353(5):476–86.

38. Czeisler CA, Walsh JK, Wesnes KA, et al. Armodafinil for treatment of excessive sleepiness associated with shift work disorder: a randomized controlled study. *Mayo Clin Proc.* 2009;84(11):958–72.

39. Schweitzer PK, Randazzo AC, Stone K, et al. Laboratory and field studies of naps and caffeine as practical countermeasures for sleep-wake problems associated with night work. *Sleep*. 2006;29(1):39–50.

40. Laudencka A, Klawe JJ, Tafil-Klawe M, et al. Does night-shift work induce apnea events in obstructive sleep apnea patients? *J Physiol Pharmacol*. 2007;58 Suppl 5(Pt 1):345–7.

41. Harvey AG. Sleep and circadian rhythms in bipolar disorder: seeking synchrony, harmony, and regulation. *Am J Psychiatry*. 2008;165(7):820–9.

42. Terman M, Terman J. Light therapy. In: Kryger M, Roth T, Dement W, eds. *Principles and Practice of Sleep Medicine*, 4th ed. Philadelphia, PA: Elsevier, 2005:1424–42.

43. Arendt J. Melatonin: characteristics, concerns, and prospects. *J Biol Rhythms*. 2005;20(4):291–303.

44. Paul MA, Miller JC, Love RJ, et al. Timing light treatment for eastward and westward travel preparation. *Chronobiol Int*. 2009;26(5):867–90.

Chapter 7

Parasomnias

Parasomnias are disorders characterized by undesirable behaviors or experiences occurring during the sleep period; the term is derived from Latin and means "around sleep." The *International Classification of Sleep Disorders, Second Edition* (ICSD-2)[1] categorizes them by the state in which they occur and includes NREM sleep parasomnias (e.g., sleepwalking), REM sleep parasomnias (e.g., REM sleep behavior disorder), or other, sleep state-nonspecific parasomnias (e.g., enuresis). There are also parasomnias that occur as symptoms of other medical or psychiatric disorders, such as sleep-related panic attacks or seizures.

Parasomnias often occur at transitions into or out of sleep, or between states of sleep. They are thought to occur as a result of sleep state instability.[2] For the brain to transition among the states of waking, NREM sleep, and REM sleep, multiple neural systems need to change patterns of activity in concert. When these transitions do not occur in a coordinated fashion, intermediate states can occur that share features of both sleep and wakefulness. Examples of these mixed states are confusional arousals or sleepwalking, which include components of NREM sleep and wakefulness, or REM sleep behavior disorder, which shares components of REM sleep and wakefulness. Individuals may exhibit several different types of parasomnias, sometimes even on the same night, or appearing at different times in their lives.

Behaviors that occur during parasomnias can range from the mundane to the bizarre, but they often represent innate behaviors necessary for survival, such as movement, aggression/defensive behavior, eating, and even sex. It has been suggested that the central pattern generators located in more primitive, subcortical regions of the brain responsible for organizing these "instinctual" behaviors are released from inhibition by higher cortical regions during admixed states of sleep and waking, thus producing parasomnias.[3]

NREM Sleep Parasomnias

The parasomnias associated with NREM sleep tend to arise from slow-wave sleep and are considered disorders of partial or incomplete arousal from sleep. These disorders typically arise in childhood, when slow-wave sleep amounts are greatest, but they are also seen in adults, often as a continuation of a childhood-onset parasomnia; the prevalence is much greater in children, however. They are most likely to occur during the first hours of sleep, when slow-wave sleep is most prominent, but can arise from other NREM stages and at other times during the sleep cycle, such as at the moment of waking in the case of sleep drunkenness.

A common feature of parasomnias is that the individual may have little or no recollection of the events the next day. Subjects are usually difficult to fully awaken in the midst of an episode, despite the fact that they may appear highly aroused or even agitated.

Factors that increase slow-wave sleep propensity, including sleep deprivation or fever, can precipitate or exacerbate these parasomnias. Anxiety or emotional stress can also increase the frequency of episodes in children and adults.[4] In adults, parasomnias can be triggered by a variety of medications, including sedative/hypnotics, benzodiazepines, antihistamines, lithium, antidepressants, antipsychotics, and others that may increase arousal threshold and/or slow-wave sleep; conditions such as pregnancy; or primary sleep disorders such as apnea or periodic limb movements.[5] It has generally been assumed that alcohol use may exacerbate sleepwalking and other parasomnias, but there is currently no direct evidence that alcohol ingestion triggers these episodes.[6] Excessive alcohol ingestion can lead to complex behaviors and amnesia during sleep, but this may represent intoxicated behavior rather than a slow-wave sleep parasomnia. Low doses of alcohol might contribute to parasomnia episodes by increasing slow-wave sleep and arousal threshold, however.[5] The association of parasomnias with psychopathology has been controversial, but some epidemiological studies in adults have suggested that they may be more prevalent in those with psychiatric disorders, particularly mood and anxiety disorders.[7,8] Often there is a family history of the same or a related type of parasomnia. Factors that are associated with an increased risk for NREM parasomnias are listed in Table 7.1.

Confusional Arousals

Description

Confusional arousals may occur during the sleep period or at the end of the sleep period; they may occur during a spontaneous arousal or following an attempt to be woken up by an alarm or another individual, but are more likely during periods of slow-wave sleep. Although appearing to be awake, the individual is typically confused and disoriented, does not respond appropriately to the situation, and may become agitated and violent, with little or no recollection of the episode. Behaviors may range from simple motor activity and vocalization to more complex behaviors, including sleep-related sexual behavior or even violence. "Sleepsex" or "sexsomnia" may be characterized by sexual behavior that is not typical for the individual, including masturbatory activity or forced sexual activity with a bed partner. More complex confusional arousals may occur in combination with sleep terrors and sleepwalking and can result in behaviors such as sleep-related driving of an automobile.

Sleep drunkenness is a type of confusional arousal that typically occurs upon attempting to waken in the morning or following a nap. It is caused by sleep inertia, with a resulting difficulty in becoming fully alert and responsive to the environment.

Table 7.1 Factors Associated with Increased Risk for NREM Parasomnias[4,5]

- Family history of parasomnia
- Sleep deprivation
- Fever
- Menstruation or pregnancy
- Stressful events
- Psychiatric disorder (adults)
- Sleep disorders
  - Sleep related breathing disorders
  - Sleep related movement disorders
  - Acute treatment of sleep apnea with CPAP (resulting in SWS increase)
- Sensory stimulation leading to partial arousal
  - Noise
  - Touch
- Medications (in alphabetical order)
  - Anticonvulsants
  - Antidepressants (SSRIs, SNRIs, tricyclics)
  - Antihistamines
  - Antipsychotics (typical and atypical)
  - Benzodiazepines
  - Beta blockers (propranolol)
  - Gamma-hydroxybutyrate (sodium oxybate)
  - Lithium
  - Non-benzodiazepine hypnotics (e.g., zolpidem)

Sources:

Mahowald MW, Schenck CH. Non-rapid eye movement sleep parasomnias. *Neurol Clin.* 2005 Nov;23(4):1077–106.

Pressman MR. Factors that predispose, prime and precipitate NREM parasomnias in adults: clinical and forensic implications. *Sleep Med Rev.* 2007 Feb;11(1):5–30; discussion 1–3.

Epidemiology

Confusional arousals are common in young children, who typically have large amounts of slow-wave sleep. The prevalence in adults is about 4% and decreases with age; men and women are equally affected.[8]

Sleepwalking (Somnambulism)

Description

Sleepwalking is generally more complex than confusional arousals but shares many of the same features, including partial to complete amnesia and a tendency to occur during the first part of the night. Sleepwalkers may be calm, and simply get up and walk to another part of the house and go to sleep in another location, or urinate in the closet or wastebasket; however, this can lead to potential danger if they wander out of the house into a busy highway or go to sleep outdoors in the middle of winter. Episodes can also be agitated or even violent, with the sleepwalker experiencing frightening dream images or hallucinations; in these cases, the individual may run from the bed and into a wall, fall down stairs, or even try to break through a window in an attempt to escape from a perceived threat. Rarely, episodes can result in violent behavior or even homicide. The sleepwalker typically has his or her eyes open during the episode but is not usually attentive to the environment; talking or shouting may occur during the episode. Complex sleepwalking episodes may have features of confusional arousals (e.g., sleep driving) and night terrors (with agitated features triggered by dreaming mentation).

Epidemiology

Up to 1 in 5 children have multiple episodes of sleepwalking, with the prevalence highest in younger children; up to half of children may have at least one episode during childhood.[4,9] Sleepwalking episodes decrease with age, with a prevalence of about 4% in adults. New onset of sleepwalking can occur at any age, but most adults with the disorder have a history of sleepwalking as children.[8] Sleepwalking has been associated with HLA DQB1.[10]

Night Terrors (Sleep Terrors)

Description

Night terrors are paroxysmal arousals from slow-wave sleep, consisting of a vocalization (usually a scream or shout) accompanied by intense fear and autonomic nervous system activation (e.g., tachycardia, tachypnea, diaphoresis). The individual may sit bolt upright in bed, or leap out of bed and run away from perceived danger; in some cases, self-injury or violent behavior may occur. Although there is often amnesia for the event, individuals who have at least partial recall often describe at least fragmentary dream imagery, usually of a frightening nature. Children may cry and be inconsolable for some time following an episode. The disorder thus overlaps in its features with agitated sleepwalking, and can occur with sleepwalking and/or confusional arousals.

Epidemiology

Night terrors are also quite common in preadolescent children.[11] There are no gender differences, and prevalence decreases with age (about 2% in adults).[8]

Evaluation and Diagnosis

Diagnosis of a NREM parasomnia is usually made by clinical history, but further evaluation including polysomnography may be warranted in cases that are potentially dangerous or disruptive to the patient, bed partner, or family members; in those accompanied by excessive daytime sleepiness or atypical features (e.g., not restricted to the first part of the night); where there is suspicion of other sleep disorders such as sleep-related breathing or movement disorders; or in cases that arise in adults without a history of episodes in childhood. Studies have suggested that sleep disorders such as sleep apnea and sleep-related movement disorders are highly prevalent in both children and adults with parasomnias;[12,13] not only can these other sleep disorders trigger parasomnia events, but also treatment of sleep apnea or restless legs/periodic limb movements can lead to improvement or resolution of the NREM parasomnia. An extended EEG montage should be used to assess possible sleep-related seizures, and video monitoring and recording is useful to observe behavior during events. Unfortunately, a patient with a NREM parasomnia will not reliably have an episode in the sleep laboratory, particularly if the events are sporadic, and more than one night of recording may be needed in some cases. However, even in the absence of an episode, sleep testing is useful to rule out other sleep disorders that may contribute to arousals and precipitate episodes (e.g., sleep apnea, periodic limb movements) and to assess for possible sleep-related epilepsy. Adults with parasomnias should also be screened for possible psychiatric disorders.

The differential diagnosis of the parasomnias described above includes nocturnal seizures, obstructive sleep apnea, nocturnal panic attacks, and REM sleep behavior disorder. Psychiatric disorders such as dissociative states or malingering may also present with similar features. Table 7.2 describes the clinical features of parasomnias and disorders that may present with similar symptoms. Guidelines for the evaluation of parasomnias are provided in Table 7.3.

Treatment

Treatment of NREM parasomnias should include attention to good sleep hygiene and avoidance of sleep deprivation and substance use. The sleeping environment must be assessed for safety; the bedroom should not contain furniture or objects that could be dangerous during an episode and patients should be protected as much as possible from conditions that might lead to injury, such as falling down stairs or wandering out of the house. Alarm systems may be helpful for patients who tend to leave their rooms or their residence. Children with parasomnias should not sleep in bunk beds. Factors that may trigger episodes should be eliminated; this includes treating comorbid sleep disorders, particularly sleep apnea and sleep-related movement disorders. Medications that may be contributing to parasomnia symptoms should be decreased or eliminated if possible.

In mild cases, education and reassurance may be adequate; this is particularly true for children, who can usually be managed with sleep hygiene and maintaining a safe sleep environment. Most childhood cases will resolve spontaneously during adolescence.

More severe cases, including patients with frequent episodes, potential injury, and/or daytime symptoms, may require additional treatment. However, there have not been appropriate clinical trials of medications for NREM sleep parasomnias and there are no medications specifically approved by the FDA for the treatment of these disorders. Many different medications have been used, including benzodiazepines, tricyclic antidepressants, trazodone, paroxetine, and other SSRIs.[15] Benzodiazepines are most commonly used and may help to decrease the occurrence of NREM sleep parasomnias by decreasing slow-wave sleep and increasing arousal threshold. Treating other primary sleep disorders that increase arousals during sleep and potentially trigger parasomnias (e.g., sleep apnea or sleep-related movement disorders) may help decrease the

Table 7.2 Clinical Features of Parasomnias and Other Disorders Causing Paroxysmal Arousals from Sleep

Disorder	Symptoms	Peak age of Incidence	Sleep stage	Time of occurrence	Confusion during episode	Amnesia for episode	Triggered by arousal	Family history
Confusional arousals	Confusion, disorientation, inappropriate behavior, possible agitation/violence	Childhood	N2, N3	Anytime, most common early in sleep period. May occur upon awakening at end of sleep period.	+	+	+	+
Sleepwalking	Walking around, disorientation, inappropriate behavior, may be calm or agitated	Childhood	N3. Infrequently N2	First part of night	+	+	+	+
Sleep terrors	Arousal from sleep accompanied by scream or shout, intense fear, increased autonomic activity	Childhood	N3	First part of night	+	+	+	+
REM sleep behavior disorder	Abnormal behaviors (shouting, kicking, punching)	Males older than 50	REM sleep	Any time of night, more common later in night, may be multiple episodes	If patient awakens, usually alert and reports dream congruent with behaviors	+/−	−	?
Sleep-related eating disorder	Involuntary eating/drinking episodes, often of items not typically eaten by subject or inappropriate or non-food items	Young adults, predominantly women	N2, N3	Any time of night, may be multiple episodes	+	+	+	+

Nightmares	Disturbing dreams leading to arousal, often accompanied by anxiety/fear. Often associated with PTSD.	Childhood; in adults more common in women	REM; may occur in N2 in PTSD	More common in latter part of night	N/A	–	–	–
Nocturnal frontal lobe epilepsy	Complex motor events, may include dystonic or hypertonic posturing, stereotypic movements, agitation, confusion	Adolescence, adulthood; more common in men	N2, N3	Throughout night, may have multiple episodes	–	+/–	–	+ in familial subtype (autosomal dominant transmission)
Panic attacks	Waking abruptly with intense autonomic arousal, including symptoms of fear, tachycardia, sweating, shortness of breath/choking, derealization, or GI upset	Adolescence, early adulthood; more common in women.	N2, early N3	First part of night	–	–	–	+; often a history of daytime panic attacks in patient
Dissociative disorder	Various behaviors similar to parasomnias, including walking around, inappropriate or agitated behavior, violence, confusion, inappropriate eating, etc.	Unknown; seen in children and adults. More common in women. Usually seen in those with severe psychiatric illness.	Waking	Any time during the night	+	+	?	–

Table 7.3 Evaluation of Parasomnias[14]

- Clinical history
  - Describe behavior in detail
  - Age of onset
  - Time of occurrence at night
  - Frequency
  - Regularity
  - Duration of episode
- Neurologic examination and EEG (including recording of wakefulness and sleep) for patients with suspected seizures
- Polysomnography should include extended, bilateral EEG montage, upper and lower limb EMG, and video recording in the following cases:
  - Paroxysmal arousals thought to be seizures when standard EEG inconclusive
  - Violent or potentially injurious sleep-related behaviors
  - Unusual or atypical features (e.g., age of onset, nature of behaviors, timing or frequency of episodes)
  - Forensic considerations
  - Parasomnias nonresponsive to treatment
- Polysomnography not indicated for uncomplicated, non-injurious parasomnias with clear-cut diagnosis

Source: Kushida CA, Littner MR, Morgenthaler T, et al. Practice parameters for the indications for polysomnography and related procedures: an update for 2005. *Sleep.* 2005 Apr 1;28(4):499–521.

frequency of parasomnia episodes. Drugs used for the treatment of parasomnias are listed in Table 7.4. Cognitive behavior therapy or self-hypnosis may also be helpful. Table 7.5 provides general treatment guidelines for parasomnias.

REM Sleep Parasomnias

REM sleep behavior disorder

Description

REM sleep behavior disorder (RBD) occurs when physiological muscle atonia is not maintained during REM sleep, resulting in dream enactment. Episodes are often intense or even violent, paroxysmal events that can frequently result in injury to the patient or bed partner. They typically consist of motor behaviors such as kicking, running, punching, crawling, sitting up, or running out of bed. Talking, shouting, swearing, or other verbal behavior may also accompany the episode. Behaviors usually involve fighting off a perceived threat, and if awakened, the individual will report having a dream, usually of a threatening or violent nature. Since RBD occurs during REM sleep, episodes are more common in the latter part of the night and usually do not occur until at least 60 to 90 minutes into the sleep period. In narcoleptics with early onset of REM sleep, however, they may occur earlier in the night. Episodes may occur sporadically but in severe cases may occur up to several times per night, corresponding to

Table 7.4 Drugs for Parasomnia

Drug	Starting Dose and Usual Range (mg)	Maximal Dose (mg)	Half-life (h)	Peak Plasma Levels (h after admin)	Side Effects	Comments
Clonazepam	0.25–2 mg qhs	4 mg/day (divided doses)	30–40	1–4	Headache, ataxia, abnormal coordination, somnolence, nasal congestion, depression, CNS depression	Used for NREM parasomnias, RBD. Other benzodiazepines or hypnotics may also be used for NREM sleep parasomnias if shorter-acting agents needed to minimize side effects. See Table 3.10.
Melatonin	3–12	Unknown	< 1	0.5–1	Daytime sleepiness, dizziness, headaches, GI discomfort, nightmares, hallucinations, allergic reactions	RBD
Prazosin	1–10 mg qhs (larger doses may be divided)	20	2–3	3	Dizziness, headache, drowsiness, weakness, palpitations, nausea, hypotension, syncope	Nightmares (PTSD)

Table 7.5 General Treatment of Parasomnias

- Assess sleep hygiene. Avoid sleep deprivation, shift work.
- Ensure safe sleeping environment. Remove items/furniture from bedroom that may result in accidents during episodes. Secure windows and doors. Protect patient from potential to fall down stairs or leave residence during episodes.
- Eliminate medications or substances that may be contributory.
- Consider medications and behavioral treatment.
- Educate members of family/household about disorder and appropriate interventions if possible.

REM sleep episodes. RBD can also co-occur with NREM parasomnias such as sleepwalking and night terrors.[16]

Epidemiology

The prevalence of RBD has been estimated at up to 0.5% of the general population.[1] It generally occurs after age 50 and prevalence increases with age, but it can appear at any age, including in young children.[17] About 90% of cases are seen in men.

RBD is usually a chronic condition and is frequently associated with neurological or neurodegenerative conditions. In studies of narcoleptics, about one third to over one half of patients were found to show evidence of increased motor activity in REM sleep and/or meet criteria for RBD.[18,19] RBD in narcoleptics may be seen in younger patients. Male predominance is less extreme for this age group; therefore, younger patients and/or women with RBD should be assessed for possible narcolepsy.

RBD is strongly associated with alpha synucleinopathies such as Parkinson's disease, Lewy body dementia, and multiple system atrophy.[20] RBD has been observed in 15% to 46% of patients with Parkinson's disease and the prevalence may be higher in other synucleinopathies.[21] Furthermore, RBD appears to be an important predictive factor for neurodegenerative disorders in that patients with idiopathic cases have a significant risk for developing synucleinopathies or dementia; prospective studies have suggested that the majority of patients with RBD will eventually develop one of these disorders, sometimes many years after the onset of RBD. Narcoleptics with RBD, however, do not appear to have an increased risk for developing neurodegenerative disorders.

RBD may also occur as an acute disorder triggered by medication use or withdrawal. Use of antidepressants (tricyclics, MAO inhibitors, mirtazapine, SSRIs, and SNRIs), caffeine, anticholinergic agents (e.g., biperiden), and selegiline have been associated with onset of acute RBD, as has withdrawal from agents such as alcohol or barbiturates.[22]

Evaluation and Diagnosis

Individuals at increased risk for RBD, including patients with narcolepsy, Parkinson's or related disorders, and other neurodegenerative disorders, and the elderly, should be screened for the disorder by inquiring about any unusual behaviors during sleep. RBD should be considered in any patient who presents with violent or injurious behaviors during sleep.

Evaluation should include overnight polysomnography with EMG leads on the arms as well as the legs to detect increased activity in REM sleep, and an increased number of EEG leads to detect possible sleep-related seizures, another cause of sleep-related injury. Diagnosis of RBD requires the presence of increased amounts and/or sustained increase in submental EMG or increased limb EMG twitching during REM sleep on polysomnography in the absence of epileptiform activity in the EEG. Clinically, patients must also have a history of injurious or potentially injurious or disruptive behaviors during sleep or abnormal behaviors in REM sleep documented during a sleep laboratory study.

Patients with RBD should be further evaluated for associated disorders. If narcolepsy is suspected, MSLT testing should be performed. Patients with apparently idiopathic RBD should undergo careful neurological evaluation for neurodegenerative disorders, including possible neuroimaging studies.

Treatment[22]

Given the risk for self-injury or injury to the bed partner, ensuring a safe sleeping environment is of utmost importance. Even with adequate pharmacotherapy, breakthrough episodes may occur. Items that could cause harm, such as furniture near the bed, should be removed. The area around the bed should be padded, and beds should preferably be low to the ground. Bed partners may benefit from protection by a soft barrier.

Fortunately, medications are often quite effective in minimizing episodes.[23] Clonazepam is the most commonly used medication, and it reduces both dream intensity and acting-out behaviors; long-term follow-up of patients demonstrated continued efficacy for a mean of 3.5 years without development of tolerance.[24] Melatonin, in doses up to 12 mg, has also been found to be helpful in some patients, although the mechanism for its effect is not known.

Recurrent Isolated Sleep Paralysis

Description

Sleep paralysis may occur at sleep onset (hypnagogic) or upon awakening (hypnopompic) and is caused by inappropriate occurrence of REM sleep atonia during waking. Subjects are fully conscious and are able to breathe during these episodes, which last seconds to minutes. The episodes terminate spontaneously but can also be interrupted by sensory input, such as being touched, or with extreme effort. Hypnagogic or hypnopompic hallucinations (sleep-related hallucinations) commonly accompany sleep paralysis, although they may also occur separately from the episodes of paralysis.

Epidemiology

Rare episodes of sleep paralysis may be seen in normal individuals and can be brought on by sleep deprivation. Events also seem to be more common during supine sleep.[25] Sleep paralysis usually begins during adolescence, and there can be a familial component. Estimates for at least one lifetime episode of sleep paralysis range from 6% to up to half of individuals.[26,27] Men and women appear to be equally affected, although individuals with psychiatric disorders may have a higher prevalence.

Evaluation and Treatment

Given the elevated rates of sleep paralysis in patients with narcolepsy and psychiatric disorders, individuals with repeated episodes of sleep paralysis should be screened for these disorders. For infrequent events that are idiopathic, reassurance is usually sufficient and no specific treatment is required other than reinforcing good sleep hygiene and avoiding sleep deprivation. Medications that may be considered in patients with frequent sleep paralysis include tricyclic antidepressants or SSRIs, since they both suppress REM sleep.

Nightmare Disorder

Description

Nightmares are the most common parasomnia associated with REM sleep. They are frightening dreams that cause awakenings; unlike some of the other parasomnias, the individual is usually fully alert upon awakening and is able to remember at least some of the nightmare. The most common emotions in nightmares are fear and anxiety, but subjects also report feelings of intense sadness, anger, or disgust. Autonomic nervous system activity (e.g., heart rate, respiratory rate) is usually at least mildly elevated during and immediately after the episode. Nightmares are more likely to occur during the latter half of the night, when REM sleep is more abundant.

Epidemiology

Nightmares occur throughout the lifespan and are more prevalent in childhood; virtually everyone has had experienced at least one nightmare at some point in their lifetime. Frequent nightmares occur in less than 5% of young adults, and in 1% to 2% of adults.[27] Women report nightmares more frequently than men, but there is not a clear gender bias in young children. Nightmare reports are more prevalent in patients with psychiatric disorders, including depression, anxiety disorders (particularly post-traumatic stress disorder [PTSD], generalized anxiety disorder, and panic disorder), and substance abuse disorders; this may explain the increased prevalence of nightmares in women, since they have higher rates of depression and anxiety disorders.

Nightmares can be exacerbated by a number of medications, particularly those that affect monoaminergic systems such as amphetamines, antidepressants, beta-blockers, catecholamines, and antiparkinsonian agents.[28,29] Other drugs that are associated with nightmares include sedative-hypnotics and barbiturates, as well as withdrawal from barbiturates and alcohol.

Evaluation and Treatment

Nightmares are almost always a clinical diagnosis and sleep studies are generally not indicated. Patients with severe or frequent nightmares should be assessed for possible psychiatric illness, including inquiry about possible traumatic events because of the association between PTSD and nightmares. Often, treatment of the primary psychiatric disorder leads to a lessening of disturbing dreams. Other factors that may contribute to nightmares such as medications or substances should be eliminated if possible. Cognitive behavior therapies may be helpful, including exposure therapy and imagery rehearsal.[30,31] Prazosin has been shown to be effective for some patients with PTSD, nightmares, and sleep disruption.[32]

Other Parasomnias

Sleep enuresis

Bedwetting, or voiding during sleep, is considered primary in children who have never had a persistent period of remaining dry at night. Enuresis is considered secondary in children who develop enuresis after a period of at least 6 months of remaining dry. Enuresis can occur at any time during the sleep period, including during all stages of sleep, arousals, or periods of wakefulness in bed.

Enuresis is common during childhood and is not treated prior to age 6 due to its prevalence and high rate of spontaneous resolution. About 4.5% of 8- to 11-year-olds were reported to have enuresis, with prevalence rates in boys over twice as high as in girls.[33] Enuresis is also more common in children with attention-deficit/hyperactivity disorder.

Adults may also develop nocturnal enuresis, usually related to other sleep or medical disorders. Enuresis is more common in both children and adults with diabetes mellitus, diabetes insipidus, disorders of the urinary tract such as infections, and obstructive sleep apnea, as well as in those who use substances such as sedating medications, diuretics, lithium, or caffeine. Enuresis may also be a symptom of nocturnal seizures.

Treatment of enuresis is related to identifying and correcting the underlying cause in cases of secondary enuresis. Primary enuresis in children is usually treated with fluid restriction late in the day, behavioral treatment, enuresis alarms, and medications (e.g., desmopressin or imipramine).

Sleep-related eating disorder

Sleep-related eating disorder is characterized by episodes of eating or drinking at night, usually with partial or incomplete recollection of the event. The episodes usually occur during NREM sleep and may occur multiple times per night.[34] Sleep-related eating is likely another NREM sleep parasomnia variant, sharing features with sleepwalking.

During the episodes, individuals may eat large amounts of high-calorie foods, or even inappropriate or odd foods, such as frozen or uncooked food, animal food, or items that are not food, such as kitchen cleaning compounds. The episodes of uncontrolled eating during the night may result in excessive weight gain, and up to half of patients are overweight.

The prevalence is about 4% in adults but may be as high as 8% to 17% in patients with eating disorders;[35] the disorder is far more prevalent in women, who make up about three quarters of cases. Predisposing/exacerbating factors for sleep-related eating disorder include other sleep disorders, such as other NREM parasomnias, sleep-related breathing disorders, and sleep-related movement disorders. Medications such as sedative-hypnotics (e.g., zolpidem) as well as other psychotropic medications (e.g., antidepressants, antipsychotics, lithium, and benzodiazepines) have also been associated with sleep-related eating disorder. There also may be a hereditary component.

Treatment of the disorder is similar to other NREM sleep parasomnias in that other primary sleep disorders should first be identified and treated, since this may be sufficient in some cases to treat the parasomnia. However, unlike other NREM parasomnias, sleep-related eating does not usually respond to benzodiazepine therapy in individuals who do not also have sleepwalking.[34] Medications that have been reported to be helpful include topiramate, agents that increase dopamine levels such as pramipexole or bupropion, and fluoxetine. Diagnostic criteria for parasomnias are provided in Table 7.6.

Table 7.6 Diagnostic Criteria for Parasomnias (ICSD-2)

Disorders of arousal

- Confusional arousals
- Recurrent confusion or confusional behavior upon awakening from nighttime sleep or nap
- Sleepwalking
- Ambulation during sleep accompanied by persistence of sleep, altered consciousness or impaired judgment, evidenced by one of the following:
  - Difficulty arousing subject
  - Mental confusion upon awakening
  - Partial or complete amnesia for the episode
  - Routine behaviors that occur at inappropriate times
  - Dangerous behaviors
- Sleep terrors
- Sudden episode of terror arising from sleep, usually initiated by cry or scream and accompanied by intense fear, with at least one of the following:
  - Difficulty arousing subject
  - Mental confusion upon awakening
  - Partial or complete amnesia for the episode
  - Dangerous behaviors

Parasomnias usually associated with REM sleep

- REM sleep behavior disorder
- Occurrence of REM sleep without atonia (increased submental EMG activity or excessive phasic EMG activity in upper or lower limbs) accompanied by one of the following:
  - Injurious or disruptive behaviors in sleep
  - Abnormal REM sleep behaviors seen during polysomnography
- Absence of epileptiform activity during REM sleep
- Recurrent isolated sleep paralysis
- Inability to move trunk and limbs at sleep onset or upon waking, lasting seconds to minutes
- Nightmare disorder
- Recurrent episodes of waking with recall of disturbing dream, with full alertness upon awakening and no confusion or disorientation, and at least one of the following:
  - Delayed return to sleep
  - Occurrence of episodes in second half of sleep period

Table 7.6 (Continued)

Other parasomnias

- Sleep-related dissociative disorder
  - Dissociative disorder fulfilling DSM-IV criteria is present, with at least one of the following:
- Dissociative episode recorded by polysomnography arises during transition from waking to sleep or after awakening from any stage of sleep
- History provided by observers consistent with dissociative disorder
- Sleep enuresis
  - Primary type: Patient is older than 5 years, exhibits voiding during sleep at least twice per week, and has never been dry consistently during sleep
  - Secondary type: Patient is older than 5 years, exhibits voiding during sleep at least twice per week, and has had a period of being dry consistently during sleep for at least 6 months
- Sleep-related groaning (catathrenia)
  - Either a history of regular groaning during sleep or polysomnography documents respiratory dysrhythmia predominantly during REM sleep
- Exploding head syndrome
  - Patient reports hearing sudden loud noise at wake-to-sleep transition or upon waking during the night, not accompanied by pain.
  - Episode accompanied by fright
- Sleep-related hallucinations
  - Predominantly visual hallucinations experienced at sleep onset or upon awakening
- Sleep-related eating disorder
  - Recurrent episodes of involuntary eating and drinking that occur during sleep and are accompanied by at least one of the following:
    - Eating peculiar combinations of food or inedible or toxic substances
    - Insomnia results from repeated episodes
    - Sleep-related injury
    - Dangerous behaviors occur while obtaining or cooking food
    - Morning anorexia
    - Adverse health consequences (weight gain) from eating high-calorie foods
- Parasomnia, unspecified
  - Used when parasomnia cannot be classified elsewhere or as a temporary diagnosis until a psychiatric diagnosis explaining the behavior can be made
- Parasomnia due to drug or substance
  - Used when the parasomnia symptoms are directly attributable to a drug or substance
    (e.g., acute RBD that occurs in response to medication)
- Parasomnia due to medical condition
  - Used when parasomnia is a manifestation of an underlying medical condition
    (e.g., RBD due to neurological disorder)

Adapted with permission from the American Academy of Sleep Medicine. *International Classification of Sleep Disorders: Diagnostic and Coding Manual,* 2nd ed. Darien, IL: American Academy of Sleep Medicine, 2005.

Other Disorders

Sleep-related dissociative disorder is a sleep-related expression of dissociative disorder, a psychiatric condition. Episodes occur during the sleep period but occur out of wakefulness, either just before sleep onset or within minutes of waking. Patients with this disorder usually have a history of severe psychiatric illness, usually with prior dissociative episodes during waking. However, these episodes may resemble NREM sleep parasomnias in that the individual can engage in complex, agitated, or even violent behaviors but have little or no memory of the event.

There are a number of sleep-related behaviors that are not considered to be pathological.

Sleeptalking (somniloquy) is common and occurs in all sleep stages, including brief or incomplete arousals from sleep. *Hypnic jerks* or *sleep starts* are also common in normal individuals; they occur during the transition from waking to sleep and are characterized by a sudden jerk, often accompanied by the sense of falling. In more complicated cases, they may also include visual hallucinations or auditory experiences such as hearing a loud noise, or other sensory phenomena. In some cases, they occur multiple times per night and interfere with sleep onset. Sleep deprivation can lead to an increased frequency of hypnic jerks. *Exploding head syndrome* may be a variation of sleep starts and is sometimes referred to as a sensory sleep start. It is characterized by an abrupt arousal associated with hearing a loud noise that is often described as sounding like an explosion inside the head. These conditions generally do not require treatment other than reassurance and avoidance of sleep deprivation.

Catathrenia, or sleep-related expiratory groaning, while a benign condition to the patient, can be disturbing to the bed partner or family members. It can occur in NREM or REM sleep and consists of a loud and prolonged groan with exhaling. It is not known to be associated with any significant medical or psychiatric illnesses and does not respond to treatments for other sleep disorders, including medications or continuous positive airway pressure.

A variety of medical conditions can become exacerbated during sleep and lead to arousals, including sleep-related headaches, cardiac arrhythmias, angina pectoris, asthma, gastroesophageal reflux, tinnitus, muscle cramps, pruritus related to dermatological conditions, and sweating (night sweats).

Forensic Issues Related to Parasomnias

Because parasomnias may be associated with agitated and injurious behavior without conscious awareness of the environment, there is the potential for patients to cause significant harm to themselves or others during an episode. Assault and murder cases have gone before the court system and, in some cases, there have been acquittals due to parasomnia (e.g., Ken Parks, who drove to his in-laws' residence and murdered his mother-in-law).[36] The criteria for evaluating sleep-related violence, as developed by Mahowald and colleagues, are listed in Table 7.7.[37]

Table 7.7 Forensic Considerations: Features of Parasomnia[38]

1. Reason from individual's history to suspect a sleep disorder, based on similar episodes in the past.

2. Duration of the activity is brief (minutes not hours).

3. The behavior is abrupt, impulsive, and senseless (i.e., without apparent motivation).

4. The victim is someone who happened to be nearby.

5. After fully awakening, the individual is horrified and does not attempt to conceal the action.

6. Some degree of amnesia may persist.

7. If a NREM sleep parasomnia, the action may have occurred upon awakening, usually at least 1 hour after sleep onset, or upon attempts to awaken the subject, and/or have been potentiated by alcohol, drugs or sleep deprivation.

Source: Bornemann MA, Mahowald MW, Schenck CH. Parasomnias: clinical features and forensic implications. *Chest.* 2006 Aug;130(2):605–10.

References

1. American Academy of Sleep Medicine. *International Classification of Sleep Disorders: Diagnostic and Coding Manual,* 2nd ed. Westchester, IL: American Academy of Sleep Medicine, 2005.

2. Mahowald MW, Schenck CH. Insights from studying human sleep disorders. *Nature.* 2005 Oct 27;437(7063):1279–85.

3. Tassinari CA, Rubboli G, Gardella E, et al. Central pattern generators for a common semiology in fronto-limbic seizures and in parasomnias. A neuroethologic approach. *Neurol Sci.* 2005 Dec;26 Suppl 3:s225–32.

4. Mahowald MW, Schenck CH. Non-rapid eye movement sleep parasomnias. *Neurol Clin.* 2005 Nov;23(4):1077–106.

5. Pressman MR. Factors that predispose, prime and precipitate NREM parasomnias in adults: clinical and forensic implications. *Sleep Med Rev.* 2007 Feb;11(1):5–30; discussion 1–3.

6. Pressman MR, Mahowald MW, Schenck CH, et al. Alcohol-induced sleepwalking or confusional arousal as a defense to criminal behavior: a review of scientific evidence, methods and forensic considerations. *J Sleep Res.* 2007 Jun;16(2):198–212.

7. Ohayon MM, Priest RG, Zulley J, et al. The place of confusional arousals in sleep and mental disorders: findings in a general population sample of 13,057 subjects. *J Nerv Ment Dis.* 2000 Jun;188(6):340–8.

8. Ohayon MM, Guilleminault C, Priest RG. Night terrors, sleepwalking, and confusional arousals in the general population: their frequency and relationship to other sleep and mental disorders. *J Clin Psychiatry.* 1999 Apr;60(4):268–77.

9. Kotagal S. Parasomnias in childhood. *Sleep Med Rev.* 2009 Apr;13(2):157–68.

10. Lecendreux M, Bassetti C, Dauvilliers Y, et al. HLA and genetic susceptibility to sleepwalking. *Mol Psychiatry.* 2003 Jan;8(1):114–7.

11. Petit D, Touchette E, Tremblay RE, et al. Dyssomnias and parasomnias in early childhood. *Pediatrics.* 2007 May;119(5):e1016–25.

12. Guilleminault C, Palombini L, Pelayo R, et al. Sleepwalking and sleep terrors in prepubertal children: what triggers them? *Pediatrics.* 2003 Jan;111(1):e17–25.

13. Guilleminault C, Kirisoglu C, Bao G, et al. Adult chronic sleepwalking and its treatment based on polysomnography. *Brain*. 2005 May;128(Pt 5):1062–9.

14. Kushida CA, Littner MR, Morgenthaler T, et al. Practice parameters for the indications for polysomnography and related procedures: an update for 2005. *Sleep*. 2005 Apr 1;28(4):499–521.

15. Harris M, Grunstein RR. Treatments for somnambulism in adults: assessing the evidence. *Sleep Med Rev*. 2009 Aug;13(4):295–7.

16. Schenck CH, Boyd JL, Mahowald MW. A parasomnia overlap disorder involving sleepwalking, sleep terrors, and REM sleep behavior disorder in 33 polysomnographically confirmed cases. *Sleep*. 1997 Nov;20(11):972–81.

17. Stores G. Rapid eye movement sleep behaviour disorder in children and adolescents. *Dev Med Child Neurol*. 2008 Oct;50(10):728–32.

18. Nightingale S, Orgill JC, Ebrahim IO, et al. The association between narcolepsy and REM behavior disorder (RBD). *Sleep Med*. 2005 May;6(3):253–8.

19. Mattarozzi K, Bellucci C, Campi C, et al. Clinical, behavioural and polysomnographic correlates of cataplexy in patients with narcolepsy/cataplexy. *Sleep Med*. 2008 May;9(4):425–33.

20. Boeve BF, Silber MH, Saper CB, et al. Pathophysiology of REM sleep behaviour disorder and relevance to neurodegenerative disease. *Brain*. 2007 Nov;130(Pt 11):2770–88.

21. Iranzo A, Santamaria J, Tolosa E. The clinical and pathophysiological relevance of REM sleep behavior disorder in neurodegenerative diseases. *Sleep Med Rev*. 2009 Dec;13(6):385–401.

22. Aurora RN, Zak RS, Maganti RIK, et al. Best practice guide for the treatment of REM sleep behavior disorder (RBD). *J Clin Sleep Med*. 2010;6(1):85–95.

23. Schenck CH, Mahowald MW. Rapid eye movement sleep parasomnias. *Neurol Clin*. 2005 Nov;23(4):1107–26.

24. Schenck CH, Mahowald MW. Long-term, nightly benzodiazepine treatment of injurious parasomnias and other disorders of disrupted nocturnal sleep in 170 adults. *Am J Med*. 1996 Mar;100(3):333–7.

25. Cheyne JA. Situational factors affecting sleep paralysis and associated hallucinations: position and timing effects. *J Sleep Res*. 2002 Jun;11(2):169–77.

26. Ohayon MM, Zulley J, Guilleminault C, et al. Prevalence and pathologic associations of sleep paralysis in the general population. *Neurology*. 1999 Apr 12;52(6):1194–200.

27. Nielson TA, Zadra A. Nightmares and other common dream disturbances. In: Kryger M, Roth T, Dement W, eds. *Principles and Practice of Sleep Medicine*, 4th ed. Philadelphia: WB Saunders Co., 2005.

28. Thompson DF, Pierce DR. Drug-induced nightmares. *Ann Pharmacother*. 1999 Jan;33(1):93–8.

29. Pagel JF, Helfter P. Drug induced nightmares—an etiology based review. *Hum Psychopharmacol*. 2003 Jan;18(1):59–67.

30. Lancee J, Spoormaker VI, Krakow B, et al. A systematic review of cognitive-behavioral treatment for nightmares: toward a well-established treatment. *J Clin Sleep Med*. 2008 Oct 15;4(5):475–80.

31. Spoormaker VI, Schredl M, van den Bout J. Nightmares: from anxiety symptom to sleep disorder. *Sleep Med Rev*. 2006 Feb;10(1):19–31.

32. Miller LJ. Prazosin for the treatment of posttraumatic stress disorder sleep disturbances. *Pharmacotherapy.* 2008 May;28(5):656–66.

33. Shreeram S, He JP, Kalaydjian A, et al. Prevalence of enuresis and its association with attention-deficit/hyperactivity disorder among U.S. children: results from a nationally representative study. *J Am Acad Child Adolesc Psychiatry.* 2009 Jan;48(1):35–41.

34. Howell MJ, Schenck CH, Crow SJ. A review of nighttime eating disorders. *Sleep Med Rev.* 2009 Feb;13(1):23–34.

35. Winkelman JW, Herzog DB, Fava M. The prevalence of sleep-related eating disorder in psychiatric and non-psychiatric populations. *Psychol Med.* 1999;29(6):1461–6.

36. Broughton R, Billings R, Cartwright R, et al. Homicidal somnambulism: a case report. *Sleep.* 1994 Apr;17(3):253–64.

37. Mahowald MW, Bundlie SR, Hurwitz TD, et al. Sleep violence—forensic science implications: polygraphic and video documentation. *J Forensic Sci.* 1990 Mar;35(2):413–32.

38. Bornemann MA, Mahowald MW, Schenck CH. Parasomnias: clinical features and forensic implications. *Chest.* 2006 Aug;130(2):605–10.

Chapter 8

Sleep-Related Movement Disorders

Sleep-related movement disorders are generally characterized by simple, usually repetitive and stereotypic movements that disrupt sleep (e.g., periodic limb movement disorder, sleep-related rhythmic movement disorder). They may also include disorders with predominant symptoms of the urge to move (e.g., restless legs) or muscle cramping (e.g., sleep-related leg cramps). In all cases, these motor symptoms disturb nocturnal sleep and/or produce daytime sleepiness or fatigue.

Restless Legs Syndrome

Description

Restless legs syndrome (RLS) is a sensorimotor disorder that occurs predominantly during periods of inactivity and at night. There are four clinical features required for the diagnosis:[1,2]

1. *An urge to move the legs, often accompanied by an unpleasant or uncomfortable sensation.* One or both legs may be involved, and in more severe cases symptoms can occur in the arms or other body parts. Patients often find it difficult to describe the uncomfortable sensations but may use terms such as "creepy-crawly," "tingling," "itching from the inside out," "pulling," and so forth. Pain or burning is not typical but may be reported in some cases.

2. *Symptoms occur or worsen during periods of rest or inactivity.* Both physical and mental inactivity contribute to RLS symptoms. Physical inactivity, drowsiness, or decreased mental activity can worsen symptoms, whereas increased concentration or mental activity may reduce them.

3. *Symptoms worsen in the evening or night and tend to improve or disappear in the morning.* Worsening of symptoms at night is related to an underlying circadian pattern and not simply to lying down at night. In patients with more severe RLS, the symptoms may occur during the day when resting or inactive, but a history of worsening at night is usually present in the early phases.

4. *Symptoms are relieved by movement or stretching.* Patients report a compelling need to move their legs, but the movements are generally volitional. If suppressed, involuntary leg jerks may occur. Movement, however, typically leads to almost immediate relief, which persists as long as the patient keeps moving.

The sensorimotor symptoms on their own are generally distressing to the patient, but they also contribute to difficulties with falling asleep and staying asleep, thus resulting in insomnia and decreased sleep duration. In more serious cases of RLS, sleep disturbance can be severe, and this is often why the patient seeks medical attention. Sleep complaints range from those primarily related to insomnia in milder cases to those related to sleep deprivation, such as daytime sleepiness and even sleep attacks, in more severe cases of RLS.

There are two forms of the disorder: early and late onset.[3,4] Early-onset RLS is characterized by the appearance of symptoms before age 45, slower progression, and a positive family history of RLS and is more likely primary or idiopathic. The late-onset type has a more rapid progression of symptoms and may be associated with RLS secondary to other disorders, particularly those characterized by iron deficiency.

Supportive criteria for the diagnosis of RLS include periodic limb movements in sleep or while awake, a family history of RLS, and a positive response to dopaminergic therapy.[1] The absence of these criteria does not rule out the diagnosis; however, supportive criteria are present in many RLS patients and their presence may help to confirm the diagnosis. Family history is present in at least 40% of patients, and at least 80% show at least an initial positive response to dopaminergic treatment, usually at low doses, or the presence of periodic limb movements in sleep (PLMS). RLS patients may also have periodic limb movements during waking (PLMW), which are experienced as involuntary, repetitive leg jerks that occur at rest; this should be distinguished from "fidgeting" or hyperactivity not associated with an urge to move. Like other sensorimotor symptoms of RLS, they become more frequent in the evening and during prolonged periods of rest.

Epidemiology

Symptoms of RLS may occur in up to 10% of the population in the United States and Northern Europe,[1] but clinically significant RLS (i.e., occurring at least twice weekly and reported as moderately or severely distressing) probably affects up to about 3% of these populations.[5] Overall rates of RLS are lower in other groups, including those from Asia, the Middle East, and Africa. Women are twice as likely to be affected, but this increased risk appears to be related to parity. The prevalence also increases with age. The most common conditions associated with the disorder are pregnancy, iron deficiency anemia, and end-stage renal disease. A variety of other medical conditions and medications have been associated with increased rates of RLS or exacerbation of RLS; these are listed in Table 8.1.

Pathophysiology

Although the exact cause of RLS is not known, it is thought to result from either an abnormality in brain dopaminergic systems or brain iron deficiency.[6,7] Any condition that produces a decrease in bodily iron stores can produce or exacerbate RLS, and correction of iron deficiency in these cases may result in improvement or resolution of RLS. Studies in RLS patients have demonstrated reduced iron stores as well as a decreased ability for the central nervous system

Table 8.1 Conditions and Substances That Are Associated With or May Worsen RLS

Medical Conditions
- Anemia related to iron deficiency
- Attention-deficit/hyperactivity disorder
- Congestive heart failure
- Diabetes
- End-stage renal disease
- Multiple sclerosis
- Narcolepsy
- Neuropathy
- Parkinson's disease
- Pregnancy
- Rheumatoid arthritis

Medications
- Antidepressants (SSRIs, tricyclics, MAO inhibitors)
- Antihistamines with CNS effects (e.g., diphenhydramine)
- Dopamine antagonists (e.g., antipsychotics, antiemetics)
- Lithium
- Nonsteroidal anti-inflammatory agents
- Prochlorperazine maleate

Substances
- Alcohol
- Caffeine
- Nicotine

to obtain iron from peripheral stores. Iron is a necessary cofactor for tyrosine hydroxylase, the rate-limiting step for dopamine synthesis; thus iron deficiency may lead to dysregulation of the dopamine system, producing symptoms of RLS. Although the beneficial effects of even low doses of dopaminergic agents suggest decreased functioning of brain dopaminergic systems, there is not yet solid evidence of a primary abnormality in dopaminergic function in RLS patients.

The heritable nature of RLS has long been recognized, with the majority of cases estimated as familial. Linkage studies have identified a number of loci in RLS families but have not identified a causally related gene.[8] Association studies have led to the identification of variants in several genomic regions that carry increased risk for the disorder. Ongoing studies will likely lead to a better understanding of the genetic basis and pathophysiology of the disorder.

Diagnosis

RLS is a clinical diagnosis, based on patient self-report. A single, standardized question for RLS screening has been developed by the International RLS Study Group:[9] "When you try to relax in the evening or sleep at night, do you ever have unpleasant, restless feelings in your legs that can be relieved by walking or movement?" This question has been shown to be highly sensitive and specific, and although it is not sufficient to make a definitive diagnosis, it is a good screening tool to determine which patients should be evaluated further for RLS. It has also been translated into a number of languages (e.g., the Spanish version is "¿Cuando usted trata de relajarse en la noche o cuando duerme, siente sus piernas incomodas, o inquietas y puede aliviar esa sensacion al caminar o con movimiento?").

Patients with suspected RLS should be assessed for the four diagnostic criteria as well as the supportive and associated features (Table 8.2). In particular, the frequency and severity of the symptoms and of the associated sleep disturbance should be determined and documented. The International RLS Study Group has developed a validated scale for this purpose consisting of 10 items, each scored from 0 to 4, with severity rating based on the total score (i.e., 1–10 mild, 11–20 moderate, 21–30 severe, 31–40 very severe).[10]

In cognitively impaired individuals who may not be able to report symptoms, several clinical features may suggest the presence of RLS. These include indications of leg discomfort such as rubbing or massaging the legs, holding the legs in pain, and excessive motor activity in the legs (e.g., tapping, pacing, cycling movements while lying down, inability to sit still). These symptoms typically occur at rest and at night, and with decreased activity.

Table 8.2 Diagnostic Criteria and Associated Features of RLS

Diagnostic Criteria

1. Urge to move the legs, usually accompanied by uncomfortable or unpleasant sensations in the legs
2. Urge to move or unpleasant sensations begin or worsen when inactive, particularly sitting or lying down.
3. Symptoms are partially or totally relieved by movement (walking, stretching) as long as the movement continues.
4. Symptoms only occur or are clearly worse in the evening or night.

Supportive Features

1. History of RLS in a first-degree relative
2. History of positive therapeutic response, at least transiently, to low-dose l-dopa or dopamine receptor agonist
3. Periodic limb movements in sleep or wakefulness

Associated Features

1. Clinical course with early onset (before age 45) usually more gradual; later onset usually more abrupt and severe. Course may wax and wane in some patients, including periods of remission.
2. Sleep disturbance is common.
3. Physical examination is usually normal. Decreased iron stores are common and contribute to exacerbation of symptoms.

Reprinted from Allen RP, Picchietti D, Hening WA, et al. Restless legs syndrome: diagnostic criteria, special considerations, and epidemiology. A report from the restless legs syndrome diagnosis and epidemiology workshop at the National Institutes of Health. *Sleep Med.* Mar 2003;4(2):101–119, with permission from Elsevier.

A number of other disorders resemble RLS.[11,12] However, careful assessment of the four key diagnostic criteria will usually allow the clinician to distinguish RLS from other disorders characterized by motor restlessness and/or leg pain. Some disorders that may be confused with RLS can also contribute to or worsen RLS symptoms. For example, peripheral neuropathy includes symptoms of leg pain and it may worsen RLS, but the two conditions are separate and respond to different treatments. Conditions that may be mistaken for RLS and the key clinical features that distinguish them from RLS are listed in Table 8.3.

No specific diagnostic tests are currently available to confirm the diagnosis of RLS. Sleep laboratory evaluation can document the presence of PLMS, which can support the diagnosis, or the presence of other sleep disorders such as sleep apnea that may be contributing to daytime symptomatology. Certainly, further evaluation for other sleep disorders and possible polysomnographic evaluation should be considered for patients whose sleep symptoms seem excessive in relation to the severity of their RLS.

Table 8.3 Differential Diagnosis for Conditions That May Be Confused with RLS

Akathisia

Most cases related to exposure to neuroleptics that block dopamine receptors and sometimes in relation to SSRIs. Also occurs in Parkinson's disease. Movements and the sense of restlessness are not localized in the extremities but affect the whole body.

Hypnagogic foot tremor

Rhythmic movements in the feet or toes occurring at transitions into sleep or light stages of sleep; may be seen in patients with RLS. Volitional component.

Painful legs and moving toes

Involuntary movements of the toes not associated with an urge to move, accompanied by aching in feet and/or lower legs

Peripheral neuropathy

Symptoms usually persist throughout the day, may improve at night in some cases, and include numbness and burning pain.

Sleep-related leg cramps

Usually involve calf or foot muscles and experienced as painful muscle contractions, relieved by massaging or stretching the muscle. Not accompanied by urge to move.

Sleep-related rhythmic movement disorder

Usually includes rocking, head banging, or head rolling at a frequency of 0.5–2 Hz. Does not typically involve the legs predominantly; larger movements/muscle groups involved. Usually seen in young children.

Volitional foot tapping

May be associated with anxiety; not a physical urge to move, not considered problematic by patient

Vascular claudication

Leg pain usually improved with rest, worsened with movement

Evaluation

Assessment of patients with clinical RLS should include screening for peripheral neuropathy or radiculopathy, and appropriate workup if these are suspected (Table 8.4). All RLS patients should have their iron status evaluated with a ferritin level as well as total iron-binding capacity (TIBC) and serum transferrin saturation level, to confirm iron deficiency as well as screen for hemochromatosis. For example, about 1 in 200 individuals of Northern European ancestry (the same population most frequently afflicted with RLS) have hereditary hemochromatosis,[13] so the clinician should assess for this prior to initiating iron replacement therapy. Furthermore, serum ferritin levels can be falsely elevated in inflammatory conditions, so they may not be an accurate representation of true iron stores.

Treatment

Not all individuals with RLS need pharmacotherapy, and a decision to treat should be based on clinical symptomatology. Individuals with mild cases may not require any treatment but should be monitored for progression of symptoms. Treatment should be considered in individuals with frequent (i.e., at least several times per week) symptoms that are distressing and/or accompanied by significant sleep complaints. In addition, those whose symptoms are infrequent but bothersome in specific situations, such as long car or plane rides, might benefit from intermittent therapy.

Patients with RLS should be instructed in sleep hygiene and cautioned to avoid sleep deprivation, since this may worsen symptoms. Behavioral therapies may be helpful, particularly for those with milder symptoms. These include hot baths, regular daily exercise, mild exercise or stretching prior to bedtime, and mentally alerting activities while sitting or resting for prolonged periods. Any medications or behaviors that may exacerbate symptoms, such as use of alcohol or caffeine, should be avoided if possible. In patients with RLS and depression, antidepressants such as bupropion, desipramine, trazodone, or nefazodone may be preferable due to their lesser effects on the serotonin system.

Iron replacement should be initiated for patients with low ferritin levels (<50 micrograms/L).[14] Not only may this lead to resolution of RLS in some cases, but patients with low ferritin levels are also at greater risk for augmentation from dopaminergic therapies (see below). Ferritin and transferrin saturation levels should be checked after 3 months of replacement, every 3 to 6 months

---

Table 8.4 Initial Clinical Evaluation of RLS and PLMD Patients

1. Examination for neuropathy
2. Serum ferritin level. If <50 micrograms/L, consider replacement to range of 60–80 micrograms/L.
3. Percent transferrin saturation. Levels <20% indicate iron deficiency; levels >50% suggest hemochromatosis.
4. Total iron-binding capacity (TIBC). Levels >400 micrograms/L indicate iron deficiency.

thereafter if iron supplements are continued, and/or following exacerbation of symptoms. Note that iron supplementation is not helpful for RLS patients with normal iron levels. Patients with chronic renal failure, iron deficiency, and RLS generally improve following renal transplantation.

Dopaminergic agents are generally considered as first-line therapies for moderate to severe RLS.[6,15] These include L-dopa and the non-ergot-derived dopamine agonists ropinirole, pramipexole, and rotigotine. Ergot-derived dopamine agonists (e.g., bromocriptine, pergolide, and cabergoline) are also effective, but their use is limited because they can cause fibrotic valvular heart disease.

Levodopa is effective in treating RLS, but the duration of action of the regular-release formulation is short; for most patients, slow-release formulations provide better coverage during the night. Levodopa is usually combined with a decarboxylase inhibitor (carbidopa or benserazide) to prevent decarboxylation of levodopa before it crosses the blood–brain barrier. Side effects at low doses, such as those used for treating RLS, are usually mild and include nausea, dizziness, and dry mouth.

Ropinirole and pramipexole are selective dopamine receptor agonists with full agonist properties for D2 receptors and higher affinity for D3 receptors. These agents have longer half-lives than levodopa, so less frequent dosing is required, with one dose in the evening usually sufficient. Both drugs decrease subjective complaints of restless legs, decrease periodic limb movements in sleep, decrease daytime sleepiness, and improve sleep efficiency and daytime quality of life. Common side effects include nausea, dizziness, and headache. Both of these drugs have been reported to cause sudden onset of sleep attacks in Parkinson's patients, but the risk of this is probably lower in RLS patients, in part because the doses used are generally lower and concentrated in the evening.

Rotigotine is another dopamine agonist that acts on D3, D2, and D1 receptor families. It has a relatively short half-life but comes in a transdermal patch formulation so that it needs to be dosed only once per day. It has been less extensively studied in RLS than other dopamine agonists but appears to be effective in improving RLS symptomatology. Its main advantage is that it provides a constant level of medication, thus potentially minimizing rebound or augmentation effects. Side effects are similar to ropinirole and pramipexole, along with the potential for skin irritation at the site of patch application. However, the patch has been voluntarily recalled by the manufacturer and is no longer available in the United States; it is not FDA approved for treatment of RLS.

Other dopamine agonists that may be useful in the treatment of RLS include dihydroergocryptine, piribedil, and talipexole, but relatively few studies on the use of these agents in RLS patients have been performed. Amantadine, which enhances dopamine release, and selegiline, an irreversible MAO inhibitor, have also shown some evidence of efficacy for RLS and periodic limb movements in initial studies. None of these agents is approved by the FDA for treatment of RLS.

The major issue with all dopaminergic therapies is that they can lead to **augmentation**, a syndrome that includes onset of symptoms earlier in the day, more rapid onset of symptoms at rest, more severe symptoms, involvement of the arms and trunk, and shorter duration of response to medication.[16] To minimize augmentation, the lowest necessary dose of medication should be used. Mild symptoms of augmentation may not require treatment. If it has not been checked recently, a serum ferritin level should be obtained since augmentation is more likely in the context of iron deficiency. If significant augmentation occurs with L-dopa or a dopamine agonist, the dose can be reduced or divided; alternatively, patients taking L-dopa can be switched to a longer-acting dopamine agonist. For augmentation that persists despite these measures and/or is severe, the dopaminergic agent can be discontinued gradually and a non-dopaminergic agent used instead, or in some cases patients may benefit from a combination a non-dopaminergic agent combined with a lower dose of the dopamine agonist.

Augmentation should be distinguished from **rebound**, which is the recurrence of symptoms during the night or early morning as the therapeutic effect of the dopaminergic agent wears off due to declining blood levels. In this case, an agent with a longer half-life should be chosen.

Dopaminergic agonists can have other side effects, although less common, that have primarily been described in Parkinson's patients. These include inducing or exacerbating psychosis in susceptible individuals, orthostatic hypotension, dyskinesias, or the development of pathological gambling or other compulsive behaviors such as compulsive eating or shopping, or hypersexuality.

A number of other agents are used to treat RLS, although none is currently approved by the FDA for this indication; they include opioids, sedative-hypnotics, anticonvulsants, and clonidine.[17] Opioids are frequently used to treat RLS, but relatively few studies have been performed to assess their efficacy. They may be useful particularly in patients with severe RLS and/or those who cannot tolerate or fail to respond adequately to dopamine agonists; they do not appear to cause augmentation. Shorter-acting opioids may require multiple dosing through the night, but higher-potency agents and sustained-release formulations may be needed for patients with severe symptoms and/or those with symptoms occurring during the daytime. Fentanyl transdermal patches provide continuous drug release and need to be applied only every 2 to 3 days. Opioids may be used in combination with dopamine agonists and may help to minimize augmentation effects. They must be used with caution, however, due to their potential to cause tolerance or dependence. Other side effects include nausea, vomiting, constipation, dizziness, urinary retention, urticaria, and respiratory depression, including exacerbation of central sleep apnea.

Benzodiazepines were some of the first medications prescribed for restless legs and periodic limb movements, but there have been relatively few studies performed regarding their efficacy. These drugs may act by helping to promote sleep onset and reduce insomnia associated with RLS; it is not clear whether they have specific effects on reducing RLS itself. Clonazepam has been the most widely used; it has a relatively long half-life, however, and may lead to daytime sedation. Like other benzodiazepines, it has the potential to produce tolerance and dependence. Information on other hypnotics is provided in Chapter 3.

Clonidine is an alpha-2 adrenoreceptor agonist and inhibits norepinephrine release. There is some evidence to suggest that it promotes sleep and may reduce RLS symptoms, and it is available in oral and transdermal patch formulations. In particular, it has been used in children with RLS,[18] not necessarily because of better efficacy but probably because there is more experience regarding its use in the pediatric population than for dopamine agonists. Common side effects are sedation, dry mouth, dizziness, and constipation. It can cause rebound hypertension if abruptly discontinued.

Anticonvulsants have shown some benefit in patients with RLS, possibly in those with pain complaints as well. Some potential advantages of anticonvulsants include that they do not appear to cause augmentation and that they are not associated with dependence. Some of them may also have sleep-promoting qualities (see Chapter 3), but this can also lead to daytime sedation. Gabapentin and pregabalin are GABA analogues that bind to the α-2 δ of the voltage-dependent calcium channel and have shown efficacy for reducing sensory and motor symptoms of RLS. Carbamazepine inhibits voltage-gated sodium channels, and although there were some early reports of possible benefit,[17] use for RLS has been limited by serious potential side effects of rash (including Stevens-Johnson syndrome), pancytopenia, and hepatic failure. Lamotrigine is an anticonvulsant with mood stabilization and antidepressant effects and also inhibits voltage-sensitive sodium channels. It, too, can cause rare, serious dermatologic side effects (Stevens-Johnson syndrome), but it is otherwise usually well tolerated. There are minimal data regarding other anticonvulsants such as oxcarbazepine, tiagabine, topiramate, valproic acid, and zonisamide at present.

Medications used for RLS are listed in Table 8.5 and general treatment guidelines are provided in Table 8.6.

When to refer to a sleep specialist

Primary care specialists can diagnose and treat many patients with RLS, particularly those with straightforward presentations and more moderate symptoms. Those in whom the diagnosis is uncertain, who do not respond to first-line treatments, who develop significant augmentation, or who have another suspected sleep disorder may benefit from referral to a sleep medicine specialist.

Periodic Limb Movement Disorder

Description

Periodic limb movements in sleep (PLMS) consist of repetitive, stereotypic limb movements, most commonly occurring in the legs but also sometimes in the arms. The typical movement pattern includes dorsiflexion of the big toe, fanning of the toes, and flexion at the ankle, knee, and hip joints. These movements last between 0.5 and 10 seconds and occur in a repetitive pattern, usually every 20 to 40 seconds, for minutes to hours. PLMS occur most commonly

Table 8.5 Medications for RLS and PLMD

Drug	Starting Dose and Usual Range (mg)	Maximal Dose (mg)	Half-life (h)	Peak Plasma Levels (h after administration)	Side Effects	Comments
Dopamine Agonists						
Carbidopa/Levodopa CR	25/100–50/200	50/200	1–3	2	Nausea, sleepiness, GI upset, muscle weakness, augmentation.	Short half-life can lead to rebound in the morning; augmentation more likely than with other agents. May be dosed multiple times during night because of shorter half-life. Administer dose about 30 min before bedtime. Compulsive behaviors, such as gambling, shopping, hypersexuality may occur.
Ropinirole	0.25–2	4	6	1–2	Headache, nausea, sleepiness, dizziness, hypotension, nasal congestion, peripheral edema, augmentation.	Daily doses > 4mg usually split into at least 2 doses. Administer at least 1–2 h before bedtime. Decreases prolactin levels. Compulsive behaviors, such as gambling, shopping, hypersexuality may occur.
Pramipexole	0.125–0.75	2	8	2	Nausea, sleepiness, loss of appetite, dizziness, hypotension, constipation, peripheral edema, nasal congestion, augmentation.	Dose may be divided across day. Administer at least 1–2 h before bedtime. Decreases prolactin levels. Possible antidepressant effects. Compulsive behaviors, such as gambling, shopping, hypersexuality may occur.

Opiods			
Mild–moderate symptoms			
Codeine	30–60	6–7	2–2.5	Risk of dependence, augmentation. Dizziness, nausea, constipation, urinary retention, respiratory depression.	Also inhibits reuptake of NE and 5HT. May worsen sleep apnea.
Propoxyphene	30	3.5–15	2–2.5	Risk of dependence. Dizziness, nausea, constipation, urinary retention, respiratory depression.	May worsen sleep apnea.
Tramadol	50–100	150	2–3	0.5–1	Risk of dependence. Dizziness, nausea, constipation, urinary retention, respiratory depression.	May worsen sleep apnea.
Severe–refractory symptoms			
Hydrocodone	30	3–4	0.5–1	Risk of dependence. Dizziness, nausea, constipation, urinary retention, respiratory depression.	May worsen sleep apnea.
Oxycodone	2.5–25	30	3–4.5	0.5–1	Risk of dependence. Dizziness, nausea, vomiting, constipation, pruritis, urinary retention, hypotension, respiratory depression.	May worsen sleep apnea.
Methadone	5–20	40	15–30	0.5–1	Risk of dependence. Dizziness, nausea, constipation, urinary retention, respiratory depression.	Use only in severe cases. May worsen sleep apnea.

(continued)

Table 8.5 Continued

Drug	Starting Dose and Usual Range (mg)	Maximal Dose (mg)	Half-life (h)	Peak Plasma Levels (h after administration)	Side Effects	Comments
Anti-Convulsants						
Gabapentin	300–1200	2700	5–7	2–3	Somnolence, dizziness, weight gain, edema, nausea	Higher doses may be divided.
Carbamazepine	200	1200	12–17 (with chronic dosing)	4–5	Dizziness, somnolence, nausea. Rare: aplastic anemia, bone marrow depression, Stevens Johnson syndrome, toxic epidermal necrolysis.	Check serum levels when higher doses are used.
Lamotrigine	25–250	500	25–32	2	Dizziness, somnolence, headache, nausea, rash, Stevens-Johnson syndrome (rare).	Dosage should be increased gradually to minimize risk of rash.
Pregabalin	50–450		6	1.5	Somnolence, dizziness, weight gain, edema, nausea	Higher doses may be divided.
Other agents						
Clonazepam	0.25–2 mg qhs	4 mg/day (divided doses)	30–40	1–4	Headache, ataxia, abnormal coordination, somnolence, nasal congestion, depression, CNS depression	Dose should be reduced in the elderly. FDA controlled substance- class. May produce withdrawal if discontinued abruptly.

Clonidine	0.1–1 mg; take 1/2 dose 2 h before usual onset of symptoms, 1/2 dose qhs	2	12–16	3–5	Headache, sedation, dry mouth, hypotension, depression.	May be useful in patients with hypertension. Also comes in a transdermal preparation.
Iron						
Ferrous sulfate	325 (65mg elemental iron; twice daily)	325 (three times daily)			Constipation	Avoid use in hemochromatosis.
Ferrous gluconate	325 (twice daily)	325 (three times daily)			Constipation	Avoid use in hemochromatosis.
Intravenous iron dextran	1000 (infusion)				Risk of anaphylaxis in up to 3%.	Treatment may need to be repeated since effects can decrease after several weeks. Less likely to cause GI side effects.

Table 8.6 Treatment Guidelines for RLS

General recommendations

1. Avoid use of medications or substances that can exacerbate RLS.

2. Instruct patient in sleep hygiene, including at least mild daily exercise.

3. Iron replacement therapy in individuals with ferritin <50 micrograms/L

Mild or intermittent symptoms

1. First line: Dopaminergic agonists may be used on an as-needed basis.

2. Second line: Consider anticonvulsants or opiates, used as needed.

Moderate to severe symptoms

1. First line: Dopaminergic agonists used prior to bedtime

2. Second line: Anticonvulsants (e.g., gabapentin or carbemazepine), or opiates, used prior to bedtime. These agents may be considered as initial options for patients with significant complaints of pain.

3. For severe or refractory symptoms, combination therapy may be needed (e.g., dopaminergic agent plus anticonvulsant, hypnotic if insomnia severe; dopaminergic agent plus anticonvulsant or opioid if pain significant). High-potency opioids may also be considered for cases that do not respond to dopaminergic agents or anticonvulsants, or in patients who cannot tolerate these medications.

Augmentation to dopaminergic therapy

1. If using levodopa, taper and switch to longer-acting agent (ropinirole or pramipexole).

2. If using longer-acting agent, consider tapering dose, dividing the dose across the day, or switching to alternative therapy such as opiate or anticonvulsant.

during sleep stages N1 and N2, are usually decreased during stage N3, and tend to be suppressed during REM sleep. PLMS occur in the majority of patients with RLS; in RLS patients, PLMS tend to be more frequent during the first part of the night, but in other patients they may occur throughout the night.

Some patients may also experience periodic limb movements during wakefulness (PLMW), which tend to occur during periods of rest or inactivity and at night, similar to RLS. Occurrence of PLMW is usually indicative of the presence of RLS, although the number of PLMS does not necessarily correlate with the severity of RLS.[19,20] Patients are not generally aware of PLMS unless they also experience periodic PLMW, but bed partners may observe PLMS or even be awakened by frequent kicks.

PLMS are often asymptomatic and not associated with obvious sleep pathology; they may be discovered as an incidental finding in a laboratory-based sleep study. However, in some cases PLMS are associated with arousals from sleep, indicated by K-complexes or brief bursts of alpha activity in the EEG. The clinical significance of PLMS is controversial because neither the number of PLMS nor arousals from PLMS consistently correlate with sleep architecture or daytime symptomatology. Nevertheless, at present individuals with either insomnia or hypersomnia not explained by other causes and with frequent PLMS may be diagnosed with periodic limb movement disorder (PLMD).

Epidemiology

PLMS are common and are seen in healthy individuals, with the prevalence increasing with age such that only about 5% of younger adults but almost half of people over age 65 may have an average of at least five PLMS per hour.[21] Women and men are equally affected. PLMS are found in over 80% of patients with RLS but are also seen in individuals without RLS.

PLMS are also more common in patients with other sleep disorders, including obstructive sleep apnea, narcolepsy, and REM sleep behavior disorder (RBD). In apnea patients, limb movements may also accompany arousals from apneic events, but these are not strictly considered PLMS (see below). In patients with RBD, PLMS may persist during REM sleep.

In general, increased rates of PLMS are seen in a broad range of medical, neurological, and psychiatric disorders, including those also associated with RLS.

Pathophysiology

Given the overlap between RLS and PLMS, it is not surprising that most of the conditions associated with RLS and substances that exacerbate them are also associated with PLMS. Like RLS, the etiology of the disorder is not specifically known; it may involve dopamine deficiencies in the brain and is exacerbated by low brain iron stores.

Diagnosis

The presence of PLMS must be documented in the sleep laboratory, in contrast to RLS, which is a clinical diagnosis. PLMS are determined from the electromyogram (EMG) recorded from the anterior tibialis muscles on both legs; contractions lasting between 0.5 and 10 seconds in either leg, occurring every 5 to 90 seconds in runs of at least four movements are scored as PLMS. In general, more than 15 movements per hour in adults and 5 per hour in children is considered abnormal, but many individuals with even more frequent PLMS are not symptomatic. Leg actigraphy is also starting to be used to document PLMS, particularly in research settings, but is not yet routinely clinically available. PLMS that occur during waking are not scored but suggest the presence of RLS. PLMS are also not scored if they occur at the termination of an apnea event.

Documentation of PLMS may not be necessary in patients who have RLS, since the treatment is the same, and it is assumed that most patients with RLS also experience PLMS. Sleep laboratory evaluation is generally used for patients with suspected PLMS without obvious RLS, who have significant insomnia, hypersomnia, or nonrestorative sleep, and for whom other sleep disorders or medical causes have been excluded. Patients who have frequent or abnormal movements during sleep may also require sleep laboratory evaluation since a number of other disorders can lead to abnormal nocturnal movements (Table 8.7). It is important to note that there is not a consistent association between numbers of PLMS per hour (PLM index) and clinical symptomatology, although a greater frequency of PLMS-related arousals from sleep can lead to sleep fragmentation.

Table 8.7 Differential Diagnosis for Conditions That May Be Confused with PLMS

Sleep starts or hypnic jerks

These are brief contractions of the limb and trunk muscles, often accompanied by a sense of falling, that occur at transition into sleep. They are common and not considered abnormal unless they occur repetitively and interfere with sleep.

Sleep-related rhythmic movement disorder

More common in children, this may persist into adulthood and includes rhythmic and repetitive movements such as head banging, body rocking or rolling, or foot tapping that begins prior to sleep onset and may continue into light sleep. Frequency of rhythmic movements is every 0.5–2 Hz, whereas PLMS are separated by longer intervals.

Fragmentary myoclonus

Very brief, irregular, and repetitive increases in EMG activity seen in the anterior tibialis muscles during sleep not meeting criteria for PLMS and not leading to movement in the legs

Arousals from sleep apnea

Leg kicks and/or other body movements can occur during the brief arousals that terminate apneic events.

REM sleep behavior disorder

Kicking, punching, and shouting can occur in this parasomnia, which is related to failure to maintain atonia during REM sleep. Patients may injure themselves and/or bed partner due to this dream-enactment activity.

Nocturnal seizures

Although most patients with nocturnal seizures will also have a history of daytime seizures, up to 25% of patients with epilepsy have seizures predominantly arising from sleep. May be accompanied by self-injurious behavior (e.g., tongue biting), loss of bladder control, confusion following episode

Sleep-related leg cramps

Intense, involuntary, painful contractions of calf and/or foot muscles. Although they can occur up to several times per night, they are not rhythmic. Can occur at any age but more common in the elderly, during pregnancy, following exercise, or with dehydration or electrolyte imbalance.

Alternating leg muscle activation (ALMA)

Brief, repeated activations of the anterior tibialis muscles alternating between legs, occurring at a frequency of 0.5–3 Hz and lasting up to 30 seconds, in sleep or during arousals. Associated with antidepressant use, periodic limb movement disorder.

Evaluation and Treatment

Treatment should be based on symptoms of sleep disruption and insomnia or daytime hypersomnia. Adults will usually have an index of at least 15 PLMS per hour in cases of PLMD, but individuals with even higher rates of PLMS may be asymptomatic and not require treatment. Unfortunately, a single night in the sleep laboratory may not always reflect the typical pattern of PLMS, as there can be significant night-to-night variability.

Other than the need for sleep testing, the medical evaluation and treatment for PLMD is otherwise generally the same as for RLS (see Tables 8.4 and 8.5). Dopamine agonists are considered first-line therapy and have been demonstrated to reduce numbers of PLMS.[6] In cases with PLMD causing significant sleep fragmentation or PLMD alone, clonazepam or a hypnotic at bedtime may be beneficial for some patients; it decreases arousals from PLMS but does not necessarily reduce the number of movements per hour of sleep.[22] In general, PLMD should be treated only when it is clearly contributing to sleep problems and daytime dysfunction; in the majority of patients it does not cause clinically significant symptomatology and does not require treatment.

When to refer to a sleep specialist

Patients with suspected PLMD should be referred to a sleep medicine specialist for diagnostic evaluation, including sleep laboratory testing. Ideally, the sleep specialist will initiate treatment, but stable patients or those who undergo sleep testing only may end up being followed in primary care settings.

Other Sleep-Related Movement Disorders

Sleep-related leg cramps are relatively common and can occur in children as well as adults.[23] They are characterized by sudden, intense, and painful muscle contractions that tend to occur in the calves or feet and can occur during sleep or waking; they can also occur during the daytime. The affected muscle may be sore and tender following the cramp. Generally sleep-related leg cramps do not cause significant sleep disruption or daytime symptoms, but they can be distressing when they occur.

They are more common in women, particularly during pregnancy; in the elderly; and in those with diabetes mellitus, peripheral vascular disease, neuromuscular disorders, and disorders associated with decreased mobility such as arthritis. Dehydration, electrolyte abnormalities, medications such as oral contraceptives and diuretics, and vigorous exercise are also associated with increased rates of occurrence.

Massage, stretching the affected muscle, and/or heat application is usually sufficient for treatment. Quinine had been used to treat leg cramps in the past, but its potential for severe toxicity has led the FDA to approve its use only for malaria.

Sleep-related bruxism includes grinding or clenching of the teeth during sleep. The behavior is quite common, particularly in children, and its prevalence decreases with age. It occurs in about 8% of the adult population,[24] but it is not considered a disorder unless it leads to sequelae such as excessive wear of tooth surfaces, jaw or tooth pain, jawlock upon waking, or masseter muscle hypertrophy. Other symptoms may include headache or facial pain. It is usually identified by observation of bed partners or household members, or by dentists who notice the increased tooth wear. Patients may also present with unexplained tooth or jaw pain or headache. The noise from tooth grinding may also disrupt the sleep of bed partners.

Bruxism has a familial component and has been associated with a variety of potential contributory factors, including other sleep disorders (e.g., restless legs, sleep apnea) and the use of alcohol, nicotine, or caffeine, and various medications, including antidepressants, antipsychotics, and stimulants.[25,26] Stress and anxiety have been implicated as factors, but their role is unclear.

Patients in whom pathological bruxism is suspected should have a clinical examination of their dentition and oral-facial region performed by a qualified dentist or otolaryngologist. Sleep recording is indicated for those in whom another sleep disorder such as apnea is suspected and may be helpful in patients with severe disorders or to assess treatment response; bruxism is sometimes noted as an incidental finding in patients having sleep studies for other indications.

Treatment options include use of a mouth guard or bite splint worn during the night. For patients with snoring/mild apnea and bruxism, mandibular advancement appliances are also effective.[27] Short-term use of benzodiazepines such as clonazepam or diazepam, or muscle relaxants such as methocarbamol, may be helpful to decrease bruxism.[28,29] Other medications that have been used include dopaminergic agents and clonidine.

Sleep-related rhythmic movement disorder includes a variety of stereotypic and rhythmic motor behaviors that may occur during quiet wakefulness, during transitions into sleep, and even during sleep; these include body rocking, body rolling, head rolling, and head banging.[23] The movements typically occur at a frequency of 0.5 to 2 Hz and may be accompanied by rhythmic vocalizations such as humming. They commonly occur in infants under the age of 9 months and likely represent a self-soothing mechanism. By age 5 the prevalence is about 5%, but the behaviors may persist into adolescence or adulthood. Prevalence is higher in those with developmental delay, mental retardation, or autism. In severe cases, self-injury may occur, usually from forceful head banging.

Diagnosis is usually made by clinical history, although polysomnography may be helpful in severe cases or to rule out a seizure disorder. Treatment should be aimed at promoting good sleep hygiene and preventing self-injury through providing a safe sleeping environment; in severe cases, protective head gear may be needed. Behavioral therapies may be helpful for older patients, including relaxation training and sleep restriction therapy to decrease waking time in bed. Medications that have been used include benzodiazepines/hypnotics or low doses of tricyclic antidepressants.

A summary of sleep-related movement disorders and characteristic symptoms is provided in Table 8.8.

Table 8.8 Sleep-Related Movement Disorders

Restless legs syndrome
- Urge to move legs, usually accompanied by uncomfortable or painful sensation
- Urge to move worsens during rest or inactivity.
- Relieved by movement or stretching
- Symptoms worse in evening or night

Periodic limb movement disorder
- Polysomnographic demonstration of repetitive limb movements
  - 0.5–10 seconds in duration
  - At least 25% amplitude of dorsiflexion during calibration
  - Separated by intervals of 5–90 seconds
- PLM index is >5/hr in children and >15/hr in adults.
- Patient reports sleep disturbance or daytime fatigue.

Sleep-related leg cramps
- Painful muscle hardness or tightness that occurs during sleep period, arising during waking or sleep
- Relieved by stretching

Sleep-related bruxism
- Tooth grinding or tooth clenching during sleep, with one of the following:
  - Abnormal wear of teeth
  - Jaw muscle pain or discomfort
  - Hypertrophy of masseter muscle

Sleep-related rhythmic movement disorder
- Repetitive, stereotypic, rhythmic movements involving large muscle groups
- Movements occur near naptime or bedtime, when patient is drowsy or asleep.
- Behaviors result in at least one of the following:
  - Sleep disruption
  - Impaired daytime function
  - Self-inflicted bodily injury

Sleep-related movement disorder, unspecified
Movement disorder that is thought to be associated with underlying psychiatric disorder and/or cannot be classified elsewhere

Sleep-related movement disorder due to drug or substance
Movement disorder during sleep thought to be due to drug or substance; usually a temporary diagnosis until primary drug-related condition (e.g., tardive dyskinesia) can be identified

Sleep-related movement disorder due to medical condition
Movement disorder during sleep thought to be related to underlying medical condition; may be a temporary diagnosis until medical disorder (e.g., Parkinson's disease) can be identified

Source: Adapted with permission from the American Academy of Sleep Medicine. *International Classification of Sleep Disorders: Diagnostic and Coding Manual,* 2nd ed. Darien, IL: American Academy of Sleep Medicine, 2005.

References

1. Allen RP, Picchietti D, Hening WA, et al. Restless legs syndrome: diagnostic criteria, special considerations, and epidemiology. A report from the restless legs syndrome diagnosis and epidemiology workshop at the National Institutes of Health. *Sleep Med.* 2003;4(2):101–19.

2. American Academy of Sleep Medicine. *International Classification of Sleep Disorders: Diagnostic and Coding Manual,* 2nd ed. Westchester, IL: American Academy of Sleep Medicine, 2005.

3. Allen RP, Earley CJ. Defining the phenotype of the restless legs syndrome (RLS) using age-of-symptom-onset. *Sleep Med.* 2000;1(1):11–9.

4. Allen RP. Controversies and challenges in defining the etiology and pathophysiology of restless legs syndrome. *Am J Med.* 2007;120(1 Suppl 1):S13–21.

5. Hening WA, Allen RP, Chaudhuri KR, et al. Clinical significance of RLS. *Mov Disord.* 2007;22 Suppl 18:S395–400.

6. Hening WA, Allen RP, Earley CJ, et al. An update on the dopaminergic treatment of restless legs syndrome and periodic limb movement disorder. *Sleep.* 2004;27(3):560–83.

7. Allen RP, Earley CJ. The role of iron in restless legs syndrome. *Mov Disord.* 2007;22 Suppl 18:S440–8.

8. Trenkwalder C, Hogl B, Winkelmann J. Recent advances in the diagnosis, genetics and treatment of restless legs syndrome. *J Neurol.* 2009;256(4):539–53.

9. Ferri R, Lanuzza B, Cosentino FI, et al. A single question for the rapid screening of restless legs syndrome in the neurological clinical practice. *Eur J Neurol.* 2007;14(9):1016–21.

10. Walters AS, LeBrocq C, Dhar A, et al. Validation of the International Restless Legs Syndrome Study Group rating scale for restless legs syndrome. *Sleep Med.* 2003;4(2):121–32.

11. Benes H, Walters AS, Allen RP, et al. Definition of restless legs syndrome, how to diagnose it, and how to differentiate it from RLS mimics. *Mov Disord.* 2007;22 Suppl 18:S401–8.

12. Lesage S, Hening WA. The restless legs syndrome and periodic limb movement disorder: a review of management. *Semin Neurol.* 2004;24(3):249–59.

13. Schmitt B, Golub RM, Green R. Screening primary care patients for hereditary hemochromatosis with transferrin saturation and serum ferritin level: systematic review for the American College of Physicians. *Ann Intern Med.* 2005;143(7):522–36.

14. Oertel WH, Trenkwalder C, Zucconi M, et al. State of the art in restless legs syndrome therapy: practice recommendations for treating restless legs syndrome. *Mov Disord.* 2007;22 Suppl 18:S466–75.

15. Littner MR, Kushida C, Anderson WM, et al. Practice parameters for the dopaminergic treatment of restless legs syndrome and periodic limb movement disorder. *Sleep.* 2004;27(3):557–9.

16. Garcia-Borreguero D, Allen RP, Kohnen R, et al. Diagnostic standards for dopaminergic augmentation of restless legs syndrome: report from a World Association of Sleep Medicine-International Restless Legs Syndrome Study Group consensus conference at the Max Planck Institute. *Sleep Med.* 2007;8(5):520–30.

17. Trenkwalder C, Hening WA, Montagna P, et al. Treatment of restless legs syndrome: an evidence-based review and implications for clinical practice. *Mov Disord.* 2008;23(16):2267–302.

18. Picchietti MA, Picchietti DL. Restless legs syndrome and periodic limb movement disorder in children and adolescents. *Semin Pediatr Neurol.* 2008;15(2):91–9.

19. Bastuji H, Garcia-Larrea L. Sleep/wake abnormalities in patients with periodic leg movements during sleep: factor analysis on data from 24-h ambulatory polygraphy. *J Sleep Res.* 1999;8(3):217–23.

20. Hornyak M, Hundemer HP, Quail D, et al. Relationship of periodic leg movements and severity of restless legs syndrome: a study in unmedicated and medicated patients. *Clin Neurophysiol.* 2007;118(7):1532–7.

21. Hornyak M, Feige B, Riemann D, et al. Periodic leg movements in sleep and periodic limb movement disorder: prevalence, clinical significance and treatment. *Sleep Med Rev.* 2006;10(3):169–77.

22. Saletu M, Anderer P, Saletu-Zyhlarz G, et al. Restless legs syndrome (RLS) and periodic limb movement disorder (PLMD): acute placebo-controlled sleep laboratory studies with clonazepam. *Eur Neuropsychopharmacol.* 2001;11(2):153–61.

23. Walters AS. Clinical identification of the simple sleep-related movement disorders. *Chest.* 2007;131(4):1260–6.

24. Lavigne GJ, Khoury S, Abe S, et al. Bruxism physiology and pathology: an overview for clinicians. *J Oral Rehabil.* 2008;35(7):476–94.

25. Kato T, Thie NM, Montplaisir JY, et al. Bruxism and orofacial movements during sleep. *Dent Clin North Am.* 2001;45(4):657–84.

26. Lavigne GJ, Manzini C, Kato T. Sleep bruxism. In: Kryger M, Roth T, Dement W, eds. *Principles and Practice of Sleep Medicine,* 4th ed. Philadelphia: Elsevier Saunders; 2005:946–59.

27. Landry-Schonbeck A, de Grandmont P, Rompre PH, et al. Effect of an adjustable mandibular advancement appliance on sleep bruxism: a crossover sleep laboratory study. *Int J Prosthodont.* 2009;22(3):251–9.

28. Saletu A, Parapatics S, Anderer P, et al. Controlled clinical, polysomnographic and psychometric studies on differences between sleep bruxers and controls and acute effects of clonazepam as compared with placebo. *Eur Arch Psychiatry Clin Neurosci.* 2010 Mar;260(2):163–74.

29. Winocur E, Gavish A, Voikovitch M, et al. Drugs and bruxism: a critical review. *J Orofac Pain.* 2003;17(2):99–111.

Helpful Websites for Patients and Healthcare Providers

American Academy of Sleep Medicine

http://www.aasmnet.org/

The AASM website provides information for patients regarding treatment and recognition of sleep disorders, as well as professional development opportunities for healthcare providers interested in sleep medicine. The Media section of the site offers fact sheets on drowsy driving, insomnia, sleep deprivation, and other health issues related to sleep; these fact sheets may be informative to both providers and patients. Position statements of the AASM on portable monitoring, herbal supplements, and other timely issues about treatment can help guide providers. Links to journals, jobs, and certification programs can help providers strengthen their ability to treat sleep disorders. AASM members may access forums and other resources, including Spanish translations of brochures on sleep and various forms and policies.

SleepEducation.com

http://www.sleepeducation.com/

Sponsored by the AASM, SleepEducation.com is focused primarily on patient education. Resources are provided for adults, teens, and children, including articles on topics such as "Sleep Tips for Students," "Dreams and Nightmares," and "Sleep Problems and your Child." Quizzes can help visitors determine if they are at risk for sleep apnea. Special sections on sleep disorders and sleep studies are geared toward helping patients understand their disorders and treatment measures. The forum "Ask a Specialist" highlights wide-ranging issues that affect patients' lives, such as bed partner snoring, the sleep of babies, and connections between insomnia and depression.

National Sleep Foundation

http://www.sleepfoundation.org/

This site provides educational materials for patients on good sleeping habits, sleep disorders, and the impacts of attention-deficit/hyperactivity disorder, aging, asthma, and other health issues on sleep. Advice on exercise, caffeine intake, and women's health can be helpful to patients as well. Audio and video clips as well as featured doctors' advice make the site useful to patients looking for multimedia resources on sleep.

National Heart, Lung and Blood Institute

http://www.nhlbi.nih.gov/

While not explicitly focused on sleep, the NHLBI website can provide supplementary information to help providers care for heart and breathing conditions that affect sleep. Special sections focus on women's heart health and menopause as well as sleep disorders. Information on obesity and diet may be particularly helpful for overweight patients with sleep apnea.

National Center on Sleep Disorders Research

http://www.nhlbi.nih.gov/about/ncsdr/

As part of the National Institutes of Health, the NCSDR website provides information on research, professional education, patient and public information, and guides for publicly accessible sleep research information.

Sleep Research Society

http://www.sleepresearchsociety.org/

The Sleep Research Society website is geared towards healthcare professionals interested in sleep medicine. Information about upcoming conferences, training, and education is provided.

Sites for Particular Sleep Disorders

American Sleep Apnea Association: http://sleepapnea.org/

Narcolepsy Network: http://www.narcolepsynetwork.org/

Restless Legs Syndrome Foundation: http://www.rls.org/

AASM Sleep Education on Sleep Disorders: http://www.sleepeducation.com/Disorders.aspx

Appendix 2

Insomnia Algorithm

APPENDIX 2 **Insomnia Algorithm**

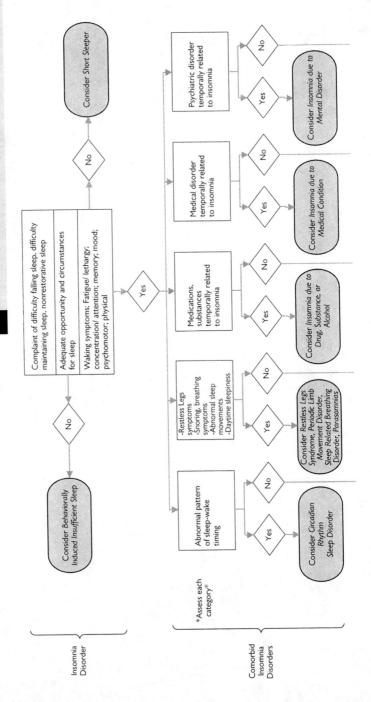

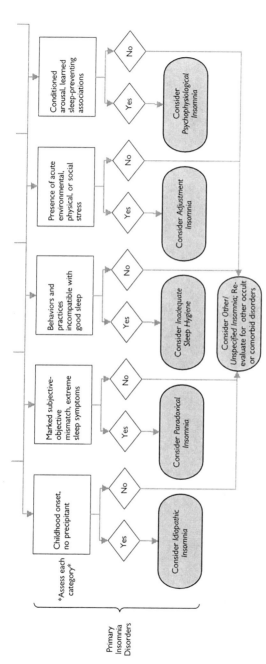

Reproduced with permission: Schutte-Rodin S, Broch L, Buysse D, Dorsey C, Sateia M. Clinical guideline for the evaluation and management of chronic insomnia in adults. *J Clin Sleep Med* 2008; 4(5):487–504. © 2008 by American Academy of Sleep Medicine.

APPENDIX 2 **Insomnia Algorithm**

ICSD-2 Diagnoses with ICD Numbers

Insomnia

Adjustment Insomnia (Acute Insomnia) (307.41)

Psychophysiological Insomnia (307.42)

Paradoxical Insomnia (307.42)

Idiopathic Insomnia (307.42)

Insomnia Due to Mental Disorder (327.02)

Inadequate Sleep Hygiene (V69.4)

Behavioral Insomnia of Childhood (V69.5)

Insomnia Due to Drug or Substance (292.85) (alcohol: 291.82)

Insomnia Due to Medical Condition (327.01)

Insomnia Not Due to Substance or Known Physiological Condition, Unspecified (Nonorganic Insomnia, NOS) (780.52)

Physiological (Organic) Insomnia, Unspecified (327.00)

Sleep-Related Breathing Disorders

Central Sleep Apnea Syndromes

Primary Central Sleep Apnea (327.21)

Central Sleep Apnea Due to Cheyne-Stokes Breathing Pattern (786.04)

Central Sleep Apnea Due to High-Altitude Periodic Breathing (327.22)

Central Sleep Apnea Due to Medical Condition Not Cheyne-Stokes (327.27)

Central Sleep Apnea Due to Drug or Substance (327.29)

Primary Sleep Apnea of Infancy (Formerly Primary Sleep Apnea of Newborn) (770.81)

Obstructive Sleep Apnea

Obstructive Sleep Apnea, Adult (327.23)

Obstructive Sleep Apnea, Pediatric (327.23)

Sleep-Related Hypoventilation/Hypoxemic Syndromes

Sleep-Related Nonobstructive Alveolar Hypoventilation, Idiopathic (327.24)

Congenital Central Alveolar Hypoventilation Syndrome (327.25)

Sleep-Related Hypoventilation/Hypoxemia Due to Medical Condition

Sleep-Related Hypoventilation/Hypoxemia Due to Pulmonary Parenchymal or Vascular Pathology (327.26)

Sleep-Related Hypoventilation/Hypoxemia Due to Lower Airways Obstruction (327.26)

Sleep-Related Hypoventilation/Hypoxemia Due to Neuromuscular and Chest Wall Disorders (327.26)

Other Sleep-Related Breathing Disorder

Sleep Apnea/Sleep-Related Breathing Disorder, Unspecified (327.20)

Hypersomnias of Central Origin Not Due to a Circadian Rhythm Sleep Disorder, Sleep-Related Breathing Disorder, or Other Cause of Disturbed Nocturnal Sleep

Narcolepsy With Cataplexy (347.01)

Narcolepsy Without Cataplexy (347.00)

Narcolepsy Due to a Medical Condition With Cataplexy (347.11)

Narcolepsy Due to a Medical Condition Without Cataplexy (347.10)

Narcolepsy, Unspecified (347.00)

Recurrent Hyposomnia
    Kleine-Levin Syndrome (327.13)
    Menstrual-Related Hypersomnia (327.13)

Idiopathic Hypersomnia With Long Sleep Time (327.11)

Idiopathic Hypersomnia Without Long Sleep Time (327.12)

Behaviorally Induced Insufficient Sleep Syndrome (307.44)

Hypersomnia Due to Medical Condition (327.14)

Hypersomnia Due to Drug or Substance (292.85) (alcohol: 291.82)

Hypersomnia Not Due to Substance or Known Physiological Condition (Nonorganic Hypersomnia, NOS) (327.15)

Physiological (Organic) Hypersomnia, Unspecified (Organic Hypersomnia, NOS) (327.10)

Circadian Rhythm Sleep Disorders

Circadian Rhythm Sleep Disorder, Delayed Sleep Phase Type (Delayed Sleep Phase Disorder) (327.31)

Circadian Rhythm Sleep Disorder, Advanced Sleep Phase Type (Advanced Sleep Phase Disorder) (327.32)

Circadian Rhythm Sleep Disorder, Irregular Sleep-Wake Type (Irregular Sleep-Wake Rhythm) (327.33)

Circadian Rhythm Sleep Disorder, Free-Running Type (Nonentrained Type) (327.34)

Circadian Rhythm Sleep Disorder, Jet Lag Type (Jet Lag Disorder) (327.35)

Circadian Rhythm Sleep Disorder, Shift Work Type (Shift Work Disorder) (327.36)

Circadian Rhythm Sleep Disorder Due to Medical Condition (327.37)

Other Circadian Rhythm Sleep Disorder (Circadian Rhythm Disorder, NOS) (327.39)

Other Circadian Rhythm Sleep Disorder Due to Drug or Substance (drug: 292.85)

Parasomnias

Disorders of Arousal (From NREM Sleep)

Confusional Arousals (327.41)

Sleepwalking (307.46)

Sleep Terrors (307.46)

Parasomnias Usually Associated With REM Sleep

REM Sleep Behavior Disorder (Including Parasomnia Overlap Disorder and Status Dissociatus) (327.42)

Recurrent Isolated Sleep Paralysis (327.43)

Nightmare Disorder (307.47)

Other Parasomnias

Sleep-Related Dissociative Disorders (300.15)

Sleep Enuresis (788.36)

Sleep-Related Groaning (Catathrenia) (327.49)

Exploding Head Syndrome (327.49)

Sleep-Related Hallucinations (368.16)

Sleep-Related Eating Disorder (327.49)

Parasomnia, Unspecified (327.40)

Parasomnia Due to Drug or Substance (292.85) (alcohol: 291.82)

Parasomnia Due to Medical Condition (324.44)

Sleep-Related Movement Disorders

Restless Legs Syndrome (333.94)

Periodic Limb Movement Disorder (327.51)

Sleep-Related Leg Cramps (327.52)

Sleep-Related Bruxism (327.53)

Sleep-Related Rhythmic Movement Disorder (327.59)

Sleep-Related Movement Disorder, Unspecified (327.59)

Sleep-Related Movement Disorder Due to Drug or Substance (327.59)

Sleep-Related Movement Disorder Due to Medical Condition (327.59)

Other Sleep Disorder

Physiological (Organic) Sleep Disorder, Unspecified (327.8)

Environmental Sleep Disorder (307.48)

Fatal Familial Insomnia (046.72)

Adapted with permission from the American Academy of Sleep Medicine. International Classification of Sleep Disorders: Diagnostic and Coding Manual. 2nd ed. Darien, IL: *American Academy of Sleep Medicine*; 2005.

Berlin Questionnaire for Sleep Apnea

Height (m) _____ Weight (kg) _____ Age _____ Sex: _____ Occupation _____

Please choose the correct response to each question.

CATEGORY 1

1. **Do you snore?**

   ☐ a. Yes

   ☐ b. No

   ☐ c. Don't know

If you snore:

2. **Your snoring is:**

   ☐ a. Slightly louder than breathing

   ☐ b. As loud as talking

   ☐ c. Louder than talking

   ☐ d. Very loud—can be heard in adjacent rooms

3. **How often do you snore?**

   ☐ a. Nearly every day

   ☐ b. 3 or 4 times a week

   ☐ c. 1 or 2 times a week

   ☐ d. 1 or 2 times a month

   ☐ e. Never or nearly never

4. **Has your snoring ever bothered other people?**

   ☐ a. Yes

   ☐ b. No

   ☐ c. Don't know

5. **Has anyone noticed that you stop breathing during your sleep?**

   ☐ a. Nearly every day

   ☐ b. 3 or 4 times a week

   ☐ c. 1 or 2 times a week

☐ d. 1 or 2 times a month

☐ e. Never or nearly never

CATEGORY 2

6. **How often do you feel tired or fatigued after your sleep?**

    ☐ a. Nearly every day

    ☐ b. 3 or 4 times a week

    ☐ c. 1 or 2 times a week

    ☐ d. 1 or 2 times a month

    ☐ e. Never or nearly never

7. **During your waking time, do you feel tired, fatigued, or not up to par?**

    ☐ a. Nearly every day

    ☐ b. 3 or 4 times a week

    ☐ c. 1 or 2 times a week

    ☐ d. 1 or 2 times a month

    ☐ e. Never or nearly never

8. **Have you ever nodded off or fallen asleep while driving a vehicle?**

    ☐ a. Yes

    ☐ b. No

If yes:

9. **How often does this occur?**

    ☐ a. Nearly every day

    ☐ b. 3 or 4 times a week

    ☐ c. 1 or 2 times a week

    ☐ d. 1 or 2 times a month

    ☐ e. Never or nearly never

CATEGORY 3

10. **Do you have high blood pressure?**

    ☐ Yes

    ☐ No

    ☐ Don't know

Scoring:

High Risk for Sleep Apnea: 2 categories where the score is positive

Low Risk for Sleep Apnea: 1 category where the score is positive

Category 1 is positive if two or more questions are positive.

	Positive	Negative
Question 1	a	b, c
Question 2	c, d	a, b
Question 3	a, b	c, d, e
Question 4	a	b, c
Question 5	a, b	c, d, e

Category 2 is positive if two or more questions are positive.

	Positive	Negative
Question 6	a, b	c, d, e
Question 7	a, b	c, d, e
Question 8	a	b
Question 9	a, b	c, d, e

Category 3 is positive if the answer to Question 10 is 'Yes' OR if the BMI of the patient is greater than 30 kg/m^2. (BMI must be calculated. BMI is defined as weight [kg] divided by height [m] squared, i.e., kg/m^2).

Adapted from Netzer NC, Stoohs RA, Netzer CM, Clark K, Strohl KP. Using the Berlin Questionnaire to identify patients at risk for the sleep apnea syndrome. *Ann Intern Med.* Oct 5 1999;131(7):485–491, Table 2.

Epworth Sleepiness Scale

Name:

Today's Date:

Your age (years):

Your sex (male = M, female = F)

How likely are you to doze off or fall asleep in the following situations, in contrast to feeling just tired? This refers to your usual way of life in recent times. Even if you have not done some of these things recently, try to work out how they would have affected you. Use the following scale to choose the *most appropriate number* for each situation:

0 = would *never* doze or sleep

1 = *slight* chance of dozing or sleeping

2 = *moderate* chance of dozing or sleeping

3 = *high* chance of dozing or sleeping

Situation	Chance of Dozing			
Sitting and reading	0	1	2	3
Watching TV	0	1	2	3
Sitting inactive in a public place	0	1	2	3
Being a passenger in a motor vehicle for an hour or more	0	1	2	3
Lying down in the afternoon	0	1	2	3
Sitting and talking to someone	0	1	2	3
Sitting quietly after lunch (no alcohol)	0	1	2	3
Stopped for a few minutes in traffic while driving	0	1	2	3
Total Score:				

Thank you for your cooperation.

Instructions for Scoring

Questionnaire is self-administered. Scores >10 suggest significant daytime sleepiness, >15 suggest severe sleepiness

Reproduced with permission: Johns MW. A new method for measuring daytime sleepiness: the Epworth sleepiness scale. *Sleep* 1991;14(6):540–545. © 1991 by American Academy of Sleep Medicine.

Two-Week Sleep Diary

Instructions:

1. Write the date, day of the week, and type of day: Work, School, Day Off, or Vacation.

2. Put the letter "C" in the box when you have coffee, cola or tea. Put "M" when you take any medicine. Put "A" when you drink

3. Put a line (l) to show when you go to bed. Shade in the box that shows when you think you fell asleep.

4. Shade in all the boxes that show when you are asleep at night or when you take a nap during the day.

5. Leave boxes unshaded to show when you wake up at night and when you are awake during the day.

SAMPLE ENTRY BELOW: On a Monday when I worked,I jogged on my lunch break at 1 PM, had a glass of wine with dinner at 6 PM, fell asleep watching TV from 7 to 8 PM, went to bed at 10:30 PM, fell asleep around Midnight, woke up and couldn't got back to sleep at about 4 AM, went back to sleep from 5 to 7 AM, and had coffee and medicine at 7:00 in the morning.

Reprinted with permission from the American Academy of Sleep Medicine.

Today's Date	Day of the week	Type of Day Work, School Off, Vacation	Noon	1PM	2	3	4	5	6PM	7	8	9	10	11PM	Midnight	1AM	2	3	4	5	6AM	7	8	9	10	11AM
sample	Mon.	Work	E						A													M					

week 1

week 2

Insomnia Severity Index

Name: Date:

1. Please rate the current (i.e., last 2 weeks) **SEVERITY** of your insomnia problem(s).

	None	Mild	Moderate	Severe	Very Severe
Difficulty falling asleep	0	1	2	3	4
Difficulty staying asleep	0	1	2	3	4
Problem waking up too early	0	1	2	3	4

2. How **SATISFIED**/dissatisfied are you with your current sleep pattern?

Very Satisfied		Moderately Satisfied		Very Dissatisfied
0	1	2	3	4

3. To what extent do you consider your sleep problem to **INTERFERE** with your daily functioning (e.g. daytime fatigue, ability to work/daily chores, concentration, memory, mood, etc)?

Not at all Interfering	A little	Somewhat	Much	Very much Interfering
0	1	2	3	4

4. How **NOTICEABLE** to others do you think your sleeping problem is in terms of impairing the quality of your life?

Not at all Noticeable	Barely	Somewhat	Much	Very much Noticeable
0	1	2	3	4

5. How **WORRIED**/distressed are you about your current sleep problem?

Not at all	A little	Somewhat	Much	Very much
0	1	2	3	4

Guidelines for Scoring/Interpretation:

Add scores for all seven items (1a + 1b + 1c + 2 + 3 + 4 + 5) =

Total score ranges from 0–28

0–7	=	No clinically significant insomnia
8–14	=	Subthreshold insomnia
15–21	=	Clinical insomnia (moderate severity)
22–28	=	Clinical insomnia (severe)

Reprinted from Bastien CH, Vallieres A, Morin CM. Validation of the Insomnia Severity Index as an outcome measure for insomnia research. *Sleep Med.* 2001;2(4):297–307, with permission from Elsevier.

Appendix 8

Pittsburgh Sleep Quality Index

Subject's Initials   ID#

Date   Time

Instructions:

The following questions relate to your usual sleep habits during the past month only. Your answers should indicate the most accurate reply for the majority of days and nights in the past month. Please answer all questions.

1. During the past month, what time have you usually gone to bed at night?

    BED TIME _____

2. During the past month, how long (in minutes) has it usually taken you to fall asleep each night?

    NUMBER OF MINUTES _____

3. During the past month, what time have you usually gotten up in the morning?

    GETTING UP TIME _____

4. During the past month, how many hours of actual sleep did you get at night? (This may be different than the number of hours you spent in bed.)

    HOURS OF SLEEP PER NIGHT _____

For each of the remaining questions, check the one best response. Please answer all questions.

5. During the past month, how often have you had trouble sleeping because you …

a) Cannot get to sleep within 30 minutes

Not during the past month _____	Less than once a week _____	Once or twice a week _____	Three or more times a week _____

b) Wake up in the middle of the night or early morning

Not during the
past month _____

Less than once
a week _____

Once or twice
a week _____

Three or more
times a week _____

c) Have to get up to use the bathroom

Not during the
past month _____

Less than once
a week _____

Once or twice
a week _____

Three or more
times a week _____

d) Cannot breathe comfortably

Not during the
past month _____

Less than once
a week _____

Once or twice
a week _____

Three or more
times a week _____

e) Cough or snore loudly

Not during the
past month _____

Less than once
a week _____

Once or twice
a week _____

Three or more
times a week _____

f) Feel too cold

Not during the
past month _____

Less than once
a week _____

Once or twice
a week _____

Three or more
times a week _____

g) Feel too hot

Not during the
past month _____

Less than once
a week _____

Once or twice
a week _____

Three or more
times a week _____

h) Had bad dreams

Not during the
past month _____

Less than once
a week _____

Once or twice
a week _____

Three or more
times a week _____

i) Have pain

Not during the
past month _____

Less than once
a week _____

Once or twice
a week _____

Three or more
times a week _____

j) Other reason(s), please describe_____
How often during the past month have you had trouble sleeping because of this?

Not during the
past month _____

Less than once
a week _____

Once or twice
a week _____

Three or more
times a week _____

k) During the past month, how would you rate your sleep quality overall?

Very good _____

Fairly good _____

Fairly bad _____

Very bad _____

7. During the past month, how often have you taken medicine to help you sleep (prescribed or "over the counter")?

Not during the
past month _____

Less than once
a week _____

Once or twice
a week _____

Three or more
times a week _____

8. During the past month, how often have you had trouble staying awake while driving, eating meals, or engaging in social activity?

| Not during the past month _____ | Less than once a week _____ | Once or twice a week _____ | Three or more times a week _____ |

9. During the past month, how much of a problem has it been for you to keep up enough enthusiasm to get things done?

No problem at all _____

Only a very slight problem _____

Somewhat of a problem _____

A very big problem _____

10. Do you have a bed partner or room mate?

No bed partner or room mate _____

Partner/room mate in other room _____

Partner in same room, but not same bed _____

Partner in same bed _____

If you have a room mate or bed partner, ask him/her how often in the past month you have had . . .

a) Loud snoring

| Not during the past month _____ | Less than once a week _____ | Once or twice a week _____ | Three or more times a week _____ |

b) Long pauses between breaths while asleep

| Not during the past month _____ | Less than once a week _____ | Once or twice a week _____ | Three or more times a week _____ |

c) Legs twitching or jerking while you sleep

| Not during the past month _____ | Less than once a week _____ | Once or twice a week _____ | Three or more times a week _____ |

d) Episodes of disorientation or confusion during sleep

| Not during the past month _____ | Less than once a week _____ | Once or twice a week _____ | Three or more times a week _____ |

e) Other restlessness while you sleep; please describe _____
_____

| Not during the past month _____ | Less than once a week _____ | Once or twice a week _____ | Three or more times a week _____ |

Form Administration Instructions, References, and Scoring

Form Administration Instructions

The range of values for questions 5 through 10 are all 0 to 3.

Questions 1 through 9 are not allowed to be missing except as noted below. If these questions are missing then any scores calculated using missing questions are also missing. Thus it is important to make sure that all questions 1 through 9 have been answered.

In the event that a range is given for an answer (for example, '30 to 60' is written as the answer to Q2, minutes to fall asleep), split the difference and enter 45.

Reference

Buysse DJ, Reynolds CF, Monk TH, Berman SR, Kupfer DJ: The Pittsburgh Sleep Quality Index: A new instrument for psychiatric practice and research. *Psychiatry Research* 28:193–213, 1989.

Scores – reportable in publications

On May 20, 2005, on the instruction of Dr. Daniel J. Buysse, the scoring of the PSQI was changed to set the score for Q5J to 0 if either the comment or the value was missing. This may reduce the DISTB score by 1 point and the PSQI Total Score by 1 point.

PSQIDURAT	**DURATION OF SLEEP**
	IF Q4 > 7, THEN set value to 0
	IF Q4 < 7 and > 6, THEN set value to 1
	IF Q4 < 6 and > 5, THEN set value to 2
	IF Q4 < 5, THEN set value to 3
	Minimum Score = 0 (better); Maximum Score = 3 (worse)
PSQIDISTB	**SLEEP DISTURBANCE**
	IF Q5b + Q5c + Q5d + Q5e + Q5f + Q5g + Q5h + Q5i + Q5j (IF Q5JCOM is null or Q5j is null, set the value of Q5j to 0) = 0, THEN set value to 0
	IF Q5b + Q5c + Q5d + Q5e + Q5f + Q5g + Q5h + Q5i + Q5j (IF Q5JCOM is null or Q5j is null, set the value of Q5j to 0) > 1 and < 9, THEN set value to 1
	IF Q5b + Q5c + Q5d + Q5e + Q5f + Q5g + Q5h + Q5i + Q5j (IF Q5JCOM is null or Q5j is null, set the value of Q5j to 0) > 9 and < 18, THEN set value to 2
	IF Q5b + Q5c + Q5d + Q5e + Q5f + Q5g + Q5h + Q5i + Q5j (IF Q5JCOM is null or Q5j is null, set the value of Q5j to 0) > 18, THEN set value to 3
	Minimum Score = 0 (better); Maximum Score = 3 (worse)

PSQILATEN   SLEEP LATENCY

First, recode Q2 into Q2new thusly:

IF Q2 > 0 and < 15, THEN set value of Q2new to 0

IF Q2 > 15 and < 30, THEN set value of Q2new to 1

IF Q2 > 30 and < 60, THEN set value of Q2new to 2

IF Q2 > 60, THEN set value of Q2new to 3

Next

IF Q5a + Q2new = 0, THEN set value to 0

IF Q5a + Q2new > 1 and < 2, THEN set value to 1

IF Q5a + Q2new > 3 and < 4, THEN set value to 2

IF Q5a + Q2new > 5 and < 6, THEN set value to 3

Minimum Score = 0 (better); Maximum Score = 3 (worse)

PSQIDAYDYS   DAY DYSFUNCTION DUE TO SLEEPINESS

IF Q8 + Q9 = 0, THEN set value to 0

IF Q8 + Q9 > 1 and < 2, THEN set value to 1

IF Q8 + Q9 > 3 and < 4, THEN set value to 2

IF Q8 + Q9 > 5 and < 6, THEN set value to 3

Minimum Score = 0 (better); Maximum Score = 3 (worse)

PSQIHSE   SLEEP EFFICIENCY

Diffsec = Difference in seconds between day and time of day Q1 and day Q3

Diffhour = Absolute value of diffsec/3600

newtib = IF diffhour > 24, then newtib = diffhour − 24
         IF diffhour < 24, THEN newtib = diffhour

(Note, the above just calculates the hours between gnt (Q1) and GMT (Q3))

tmphse = (Q4 / newtib) * 100

IF tmphse > 85, THEN set value to 0

IF tmphse < 85 and > 75, THEN set value to 1

IF tmphse < 75 and > 65, THEN set value to 2

IF tmphse < 65, THEN set value to 3

Minimum Score = 0 (better); Maximum Score = 3 (worse)

PSQISLPQUAL OVERALL SLEEP QUALITY

Q6

Minimum Score = 0 (better); Maximum Score = 3 (worse)

PSQIMEDS   NEED MEDS TO SLEEP

Q7

Minimum Score = 0 (better); Maximum Score = 3 (worse)

PSQI   TOTAL

DURAT + DISTB + LATEN + DAYDYS + HSE + SLPQUAL + MEDS

Minimum Score = 0 (better); Maximum Score = 21 (worse)

Interpretation: TOTAL < 5 associated with good sleep quality

TOTAL > 5 associated with poor sleep quality

Appendix 9

Morningness–Eveningness Questionnaire

Name: _____   Date: _____

Age: _____   Sex: _____

For each of the following questions, please select the answer that best describes you. Make your judgements based on how you have felt in recent weeks. There are no "right" or "wrong" answers; just pick the answers that fit YOU best.

1. *Approximately* what time would you get up if you were entirely free to plan your own day?

   [5] 5:00 a.m. – 6:30 a.m.

   [4] 6:30 a.m. – 7:45 a.m.

   [3] 7:45 a.m. – 9:45 a.m.

   [2] 9:45 a.m. – 11:00 a.m.

   [1] 11:00 a.m. – 12 noon

2. *Approximately* what time would you go to bed if you were entirely free to plan your evening?

   [5] 8:00 p.m. – 9:00 p.m.

   [4] 9:00 p.m. – 10:15 p.m.

   [3] 10:15 p.m. – 12:30 a.m.

   [2] 12:30 a.m. – 1:45 a.m.

   [1] 1:45 a.m. – 3:00 a.m.

3. If you usually have to get up at a specific time in the morning, how much do you depend on an alarm clock?

   [4] Not at all

   [3] Slightly

   [2] Somewhat

   [1] Very much

4. How easy do you find it to get up in the morning (when you are not awakened unexpectedly)?

   [1] Very difficult

   [2] Somewhat difficult

   [3] Fairly easy

   [4] Very easy

5. How alert do you feel during the first half hour after you wake up in the morning?

   [1] Not at all alert

   [2] Slightly alert

   [3] Fairly alert

   [4] Very alert

6. How hungry do you feel during the first half hour after you wake up?

   [1] Not at all hungry

   [2] Slightly hungry

   [3] Fairly hungry

   [4] Very hungry

7. During the first half hour after you wake up in the morning, how do you feel?

   [1] Very tired

   [2] Fairly tired

   [3] Fairly refreshed

   [4] Very refreshed

8. If you had no commitments the next day, what time would you go to bed compared to your usual bedtime?

   [4] Seldom or never later

   [3] Less than 1 hour later

   [2] 1–2 hours later

   [1] More than 2 hours later

9. You have decided to do physical exercise. A friend suggests that you do this for one hour twice a week, and the best time for him is between 7 and 8 a.m. Bearing in mind nothing but your own internal "clock," how do you think you would perform?

   [4] Would be in good form

   [3] Would be in reasonable form

[2] Would find it difficult

[1] Would find it very difficult

10. At *approximately* what time in the evening do you feel tired, and, as a result, in need of sleep?

[5] 8:00 p.m. – 9:00 p.m.

[4] 9:00 p.m. – 10:15 p.m.

[3] 10:15 p.m. – 12:45 a.m.

[2] 12:45 a.m. – 2:00 a.m.

[1] 2:00 a.m. – 3:00 a.m.

11. You want to be at your peak performance for a test that you know is going to be mentally exhausting and will last two hours. You are entirely free to plan your day. Considering only your internal "clock," which one of the four testing times would you choose?

[6] 8 a.m. – 10 a.m.

[4] 11 a.m. – 1 p.m.

[2] 3 p.m. – 5 p.m.

[0] 7 p.m. – 9 p.m.

12. If you got into bed at 11 p.m., how tired would you be?

[0] Not at all tired

[2] A little tired

[3] Fairly tired

[5] Very tired

13. For some reason you have gone to bed several hours later than usual, but there is no need to get up at any particular time the next morning. Which one of the following are you most likely to do?

[4] Will wake up at usual time, but will not fall back asleep

[3] Will wake up at usual time and will doze thereafter

[2] Will wake up at the usual time, but will fall asleep again

[1] Will not wake up until later than usual

14. One night you have to remain awake between 4 and 6 a.m. in order to carry out a night watch. You have no time commitments the next day. Which one of the alternatives would suit you best?

[1] Would not go to bed until the watch is over

[2] Would take a nap before and sleep after

[3] Would take a good sleep before and nap after

[4] Would sleep only before the watch

15. You have two hours of hard physical work. You are entirely free to plan your day. Considering only your internal "clock", which of the following times would you choose?

    [4] 8 a.m. – 10 a.m.

    [3] 11 a.m. – 1 p.m.

    [2] 3 p.m. – 5 p.m.

    [1] 7 p.m. – 9 p.m.

16. You have decided to do physical exercise. A friend suggests that you do this for one hour twice a week. The best time for her is between 10 and 11 p.m. Bearing in mind only your internal "clock", how well do you think you would perform?

    [1] Would be in good form

    [2] Would be in reasonable form

    [3] Would find it difficult

    [4] Would find it very difficult

17. Suppose you can choose your own work hours. Assume that you work a five- hour day (including breaks), your job is interesting, and you are paid based on your performance. At *approximately* what time would you choose to begin?

    [5] 5 hours starting between 4:00 – 8:00 a.m.

    [4] 5 hours starting between 8:00 – 9:00 a.m.

    [3] 5 hours starting between 9:00 a.m. – 2:00 p.m.

    [2] 5 hours starting between 2:00 – 5:00 p.m.

    [1] 5 hours starting between 5:00 p.m. – 4:00 a.m.

18. At *approximately* what time of day do you usually feel your best?

    [5] 5:00 a.m. – 8:00 a.m.

    [4] 8:00 a.m. – 10:00 a.m.

    [3] 10:00 a.m. – 5:00 p.m.

    [2] 5:00 p.m. – 10:00 p.m.

    [1] 10:00 p.m. – 5:00 a.m.

19. One hears about "morning types" and "evening types." Which one of these types do you consider yourself to be?

    [6] Definitely a morning type

    [4] Rather more a morning type than an evening type

    [2] Rather more an evening type than a morning type

    [0] Definitely an evening type

Total Score: _____

Instructions for Scoring

Add up the total points from the questions. Total scores indicate the following: Definitely morning type (70–86); Moderately morning type (59–69); Neither type (42–58); Moderately evening type (31–41); Definitely evening type (16–30).

Adapted by Mary Carskadon from Horne JA, Ostberg O. A self-assessment questionnaire to determine morningness-eveningness in human circadian rhythms. *Int J Chronobiol.* 1976;4(2):97–110.

Appendix 10

Body Mass Index Table

	Normal						Overweight					Obese										Extreme Obesity														
BMI	19	20	21	22	23	24	25	26	27	28	29	30	31	32	33	34	35	36	37	38	39	40	41	42	43	44	45	46	47	48	49	50	51	52	53	54
Height (inches)												Body Weight (pounds)																								
58	91	96	100	105	110	115	119	124	129	134	138	143	148	153	158	162	167	172	177	181	186	191	196	201	205	210	215	220	224	229	234	239	244	248	253	258
59	94	99	104	109	114	119	124	128	133	138	143	148	153	158	163	168	173	178	183	188	193	198	203	208	212	217	222	227	232	237	242	247	252	257	262	267
60	97	102	107	112	118	123	128	133	138	143	148	153	158	163	168	174	179	184	189	194	199	204	209	215	220	225	230	235	240	245	250	255	261	266	271	276
61	100	106	111	116	122	127	132	137	143	148	153	158	164	169	174	180	185	190	195	201	206	211	217	222	227	232	238	243	248	254	259	264	269	275	280	285
62	104	109	115	120	126	131	136	142	147	153	158	164	169	175	180	186	191	196	202	207	213	218	224	229	235	240	246	251	256	262	267	273	278	284	289	295
63	107	113	118	124	130	135	141	146	152	158	163	169	175	180	186	191	197	203	208	214	220	225	231	237	242	248	254	259	265	270	278	282	287	293	299	304
64	110	116	122	128	134	140	145	151	157	163	169	174	180	186	192	197	204	209	215	221	227	232	238	244	250	256	262	267	273	279	285	291	296	302	308	314
65	114	120	126	132	138	144	150	156	162	168	174	180	186	192	198	204	210	216	222	228	234	240	246	252	258	264	270	276	282	288	294	300	306	312	318	324
66	118	124	130	136	142	148	155	161	167	173	179	186	192	198	204	210	216	223	229	235	241	247	253	260	266	272	278	284	291	297	303	309	315	322	328	334

67	121	127	134	140	146	153	159	166	172	178	185	191	198	204	211	217	223	230	236	242	249	255	261	268	274	280	287	293	299	306	312	319	325	331	338	344
68	125	131	138	144	151	158	164	171	177	184	190	197	203	210	216	223	230	236	243	249	256	262	269	276	282	289	295	302	308	315	322	328	335	341	348	354
69	128	135	142	149	155	162	169	176	182	189	196	203	209	216	223	230	236	243	250	257	263	270	277	284	291	297	304	311	318	324	331	338	345	351	358	365
70	132	139	146	153	160	167	174	181	188	195	202	209	216	222	229	236	243	250	257	264	271	278	285	292	299	306	313	320	327	334	341	348	355	362	369	376
71	136	143	150	157	165	172	179	186	193	200	208	215	222	229	236	243	250	257	265	272	279	286	293	301	308	315	322	329	338	343	351	358	365	372	379	386
72	140	147	154	162	169	177	184	191	199	206	213	221	228	235	242	250	258	265	272	279	287	294	302	309	316	324	331	338	346	353	361	368	375	383	390	397
73	144	151	159	166	174	182	189	197	204	212	219	227	235	242	250	257	265	272	280	288	295	302	310	318	325	333	340	348	355	363	371	378	386	393	401	408
74	148	155	163	171	179	186	194	202	210	218	225	233	241	249	256	264	272	280	287	295	303	311	319	326	334	342	350	358	365	373	381	389	396	404	412	420
75	152	160	168	176	184	192	200	208	216	224	232	240	248	256	264	272	279	287	295	303	311	319	327	335	343	351	359	367	375	383	391	399	407	415	423	431
76	156	164	172	180	189	197	205	213	221	230	238	246	254	263	271	279	287	295	304	312	320	328	336	344	353	361	369	377	385	394	402	410	418	426	435	443

Source: Adapted from Clinical Guidelines on the Identification, Evaluation, and Treatment of Overweight and Obesity in Adults: The Evidence Report.

APPENDIX 10 **Body Mass Index Table**

Appendix 11

Center for Epidemiologic Studies Depression Scale (CES-D), NIMH

Below is a list of the ways you might have felt or behaved. Please tell me how often you have felt this way during the past week.

	During the Past Week			
	Rarely or none of the time (less than 1 day)	Some or a little of the time (1–2 days)	Occasionally or a moderate amount of the time (3–4 days)	Most or all of the time (5–7 days)
1. I was bothered by things that don't usually bother me.				
2. I did not feel like eating; my appetite was poor.				
3. I felt that I could not shake off the blues even with the help of my family or friends.				
4. I felt that I was just as good as other people.				
5. I had trouble keeping my mind on what I was doing.				
6. I felt depressed.				
7. I felt everything I did was an effort.				
8. I felt hopeful about the future.				
9. I thought my life had been a failure.				

	During the Past Week			
	Rarely or none of the time (less than 1 day)	Some or a little of the time (1–2 days)	Occasionally or a moderate amount of the time (3–4 days)	Most or all of the time (5–7 days)
10. I felt fearful.				
11. My sleep was restless.				
12. I was happy.				
13. I talked less than usual.				
14. I felt lonely.				
15. People were unfriendly.				
16. I enjoyed life.				
17. I had crying spells.				
18. I felt sad.				
19. I felt that people disliked me.				
20. I could not get "going".				

SCORING: 0 for answers in the first column, 1 for answers in the second column, 2 for answers in the third column, 3 for answers in the fourth column. The scoring of positive items is reversed. Possible range of scores is 0 to 60, with the higher scores indicating the presence of more symptomatology.

Reprinted with permission from Radloff LS. The CES-D scale: A self report depression scale for research in the general population. *Applied Psychological Measurement.* 1977;1:385–401.

Index

A

AASM (American Academy of Sleep Medicine), 51, 65, 181
Acetazolamide, 88, 89t
Actigraphy
  defined, *114*
  description (parameters measured), 42, *43*
  DSPD evaluation, *115*
  for circadian rhythm disorders, 134t
  for SWD, 129
  indications, included data, 44
  ISWR evaluation, *122*
Adaptive servoventilation (ASV) treatment, for CSA, 88
Advanced sleep phase disorder (ASPD), 121
  description, 120
  epidemiology, 120
  evaluation/diagnosis, 121
  pathophysiology, 120–121
  treatment, 121
Alcohol
  excessive sleepiness and, 96
  insomnia and, 50t, 53, 54t, 56, 57, 62
  snoring and, 73, 74, 75t
American Academy of Sleep Medicine (AASM), 51, 65, 181
Amitriptyline, 63, 67t
Amphetamine/
  dextroamphetamine extended release, 109t
Amphetamines
  for excessive sleepiness, 105–106, 108t, 109t
  mechanism of action, 14
  nightmare exacerbation from, 150
Anti-cholinergic medications, 15, 62, 64, 106, 110t
Anticonvulsants, 64–65. See *also* Gabapentin
  and excessive sleepiness, 97t
  side effects, 65
Antidepressants
  for excessive sleepiness, 97t, 106
  sedating antidepressants, 63–64
  side effects, 64
Antiemetics, 161t

Antihistamines, 62. See *also* Diphenhydramine; Doxylamine
  as parasomnia trigger, 140, 141t
  as RLS trigger, 161t
  mechanism of action, 14
  negative influence on insomnia, 65t
  risk factors, 123
Antipsychotics, 67t, 69, 123. See *also* Clozapine; Olanzapine; Quetiapine
  and bruxism, 176
  and RLS, 161
  and sleep-related eating disorders, 151–152
  as parasomnia trigger, 140, 141t
  contraindications, 65t, 117t
  for insomnia, 65
  risk factors, 123
  sedating effect, 63
Apnea-hypopnea index (AHI), 80
Apneas. See Central sleep apnea; Mixed apneas; Obstructive sleep apnea
Armodafinil
  for excessive sleepiness, 105, 108t
  for shift work disorder, 130, 132t
Ascending reticular activating system (ARAS), 13–14
Atomoxetine, 10
Autotitrating positive airway pressure (APAP) treatment, for OSA, 81

B

Beck Depression Inventory, 52, 54t
Benzodiazepine receptor agonists (BzRAs), 62–63, 66t
  as insomnia first line agent, 69
  benzodiazepines, 66t
  nonbenzodiazepines, 66t
  side effects, 63
Benzodiazepines
  contraindications, 63, 78t, 83t, 87t
  for insomnia, 62
  for NREM sleep parasomnias, 143

  for sleep-related eating disorder, 151–152
  parasomnias and, 140, 141t, 143, 147t
  side effects, 63
Berlin Questionnaire for Sleep Apnea, 28, 79, 191–193
Biofeedback, 59t, 61, 61t
Body mass index table, 214t–215t
BPAP (bilevel positive airway pressure) treatment
  for CSA, 88
  for OSA, 81
Brain systems involvement
  amygdala, 15–16
  neural networks, *12, 13*
Bruxism (teeth grinding), 26, 175–176
Bupropion, 50t, 152, 164

C

Caffeine
  for shift work disorder, 130–131
  insomnia and, 53, 54t, 56t
  jet lag and, 126–127, 128t
  mechanism of action, 105
  shift work disorder and, 130–131, 132t
  side effects of, 127
Carbamazepine
  for PLMS, 170t
  for RLS, 167, 170t
Cataplexy
  evaluation, 99
  excessive sleepiness and, 98–101
  narcolepsy with/without, 98, 101, 102t
  pharmacologic treatment, 110t
Catathrenia, 154
Center for Epidemiologic Studies Depression Scale (CES-D), 29, 52, 217–218
Central sleep apnea (CSA)
  description, 86
  epidemiology, 86–87
  evaluation/diagnosis, 88
  measurements, *34, 35*
  pathophysiology, 87–88
  primary central sleep apnea, 87, 88, 89t
  risk factors, 87
  symptoms, 86t
  treatment, 88–89, 89t

CPSIA information can be obtained
at www.ICGtesting.com
Printed in the USA
FFOW01n1839180516
24167FF